Sleeplessn

Jim Horne

Sleeplessness

Assessing Sleep Need in Society Today

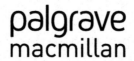

Jim Horne
Loughborough University
Leicestershire, UK

ISBN 978-3-319-30571-4 (hard cover)   ISBN 978-3-319-30572-1   (eBook)
ISBN 978-3-319-32791-4 (soft cover)
DOI 10.1007/978-3-319-30572-1

Library of Congress Control Number: 2016940600

Cover illustration: © H. Mark Weidman Photography / Alamy Stock Photo

Printed on acid-free paper

This Palgrave Macmillan imprint is published by Springer Nature
The registered company is Springer International Publishing AG Switzerland

To My Family

Preface

Apparently, many of us in today's society are, unknowingly, suffering from chronic sleep loss, known as 'sleep debt'—search the term on the internet and there are millions of hits. This 'societal insomnia' is largely attributed to the pressures of modern waking life, and seems to be yet another cause of obesity, cardiovascular disease and other disorders. Besides, such claims further add to the worries of those actually suffering with insomnia, striving even for 6 hours' sleep, only to hear that 7–8 hours is the ideal goal. Yet, human nature being what it is, little has actually changed since Victorian times, when 'sleeplessness' was a common topic of medical debate, and it is here where we begin, with some remarkable insights from physicians of that era, that ought still to give us pause for thought, and underlies the theme of this book.

A diagnosis of 'insomnia', and indeed the term itself, is largely a twentieth century convention, mostly heralded by the discovery of new hypnotic medicines, allowing the condition to become more 'medicalised' rather than a more benign 'fact of life', as it was then seen to be. By continuing to take this more 'matter of fact' approach to today's sleep debt, *Sleeplessness* looks more closely and dispassionately at insomnia itself, its various phenomena, and the 'overwakefulness' that pervades it, which is more likely to be remedied, not by sleeping tablets alone, but by the therapies of wakefulness rather than those of sleep.

Moving on to the wider issues of 'societal insomnia', *Sleeplessness* argues that sleep debt is overstated, as the great majority of us have sufficient sleep, especially as our 7-hour average sleep has changed little over the last century. Thus claims that we 'need 8 hours' are doubtful, as most of us happily sleep less than this amount and, apart from the natural differences between people in the duration of their sleep, judging it merely by its length overlooks the importance of its quality, and another underlying theme for *Sleeplessness*.

Hour by hour, a night's sleep is not equivalent in terms of its recuperation. As one might expect, sleep at its beginning, reflected by the EEG as 'slow wave sleep' (SWS—'deep sleep'), is more beneficial than sleep towards its end, when Rapid Eye Movement sleep (REM) is at its most prolific, with its accompanying dreaming at its most intense. Whilst SWS seems to be critical for the brain's (cortical) recovery following the demands of prior wakefulness, REM is much like wakefulness and mostly seems to prepare us for the ensuing wakefulness, more so with 'emotional preparedness', maybe even linked to food choice and its desirability. More to the point, REM towards the end of sleep seems to be interchangeable with wakefulness depending on whether waking needs are greater or lesser, when REM can act as a time-filler to extend sleep when the pressure for wakefulness is low, or taken simply from pleasure. Such a flexibility in sleep duration, especially with REM, and without necessarily affecting sleepiness nor a need for extra 'recovery sleep', is not achieved 'overnight' but can require longer-term adaptation. For example, before the advent of the electric light and with the seasonal changes in daylight and food availability, waking pressures on sleep duration would naturally alter, as can still be seen in today's non-industrial societies. Interestingly, REM has brain mechanisms in common with feeding behaviour, with REM also able to suppress feelings of hunger appearing towards the end of our nocturnal sleep which usually develops into a fast.

All our biological needs are flexible, harmlessly able to be reduced somewhat, or taken to excess, as with our ability to eat and drink beyond the feelings of hunger and thirst, depending on tempting opportunities from the sight and smell of attractive food, or the social drinking of coffee, tea and beer for example.

A critical examination of the links between short sleep and mortality, obesity, diabetes and heart disease, shows these to be modest at best, only really seen in those sleeping fewer than five hours a night, where many, here, are indeed chronically sleep deprived, but who comprise only a small minority of the population. Whether this inadequate sleep is an actual cause rather than a correlate of obesity, for example, is a matter for much debate, despite statistically significant findings which, in real terms, are often too small to be of real clinical significance. This issue, that both types of 'significance' are synonymous, is misleading and can be seen with other aspects of sleep and, again, all too easily leading to other potentially worrying distortions of actual risks. For example, weight gains attributed to sleep debt, even for 5-hour sleepers, typically average less than 2 kilograms a year, contrasting with those hundreds of hours of apparently annually accumulated 'lost' sleep. Besides, few obese adults are such short sleepers, and neither by extending their sleep, nor by using sleeping tablets, is any such weight gain likely to be prevented, particularly when compared with the far more rapid effectiveness of diet and exercise.

The extent to which today's children and adolescents suffer from sleep debt is another focus for *Sleeplessness* comprising similar issues and controversies. Again, the historical evidence is revealing when compared with the extensive recent findings and, once more, it is *plus ça change ...* particularly when considering obesity and the extent of the claims that this is also linked to their short sleep.

More light, especially daylight, is shed on the body (circadian) clock, both in its role as the terminator of sleep, and on the recent, popular concept of 'social jet lag' which, in many respects, is akin to sleep debt. Yet again, these factors also reflect the ability of our sleep to adapt (within limits) to essential waking needs, in a 'give and take' manner. However, as shift work and actual jet lag do present difficulties, these topics have an airing that includes practical advice.

Inasmuch as we can sleep to excess, then it is argued, here, that the sleepiness preceding this 'extra' sleep is not indicative of sleep need, but is incidental or 'situational', overcome without the need for sleep, but by more worthwhile waking activities. This is comparable with our 'appetite' for food, as in that tempting second helping, rather than hunger as in a need to eat. However, this 'appetitive' sleepiness, unnoticeable in everyday activities can be eked out by boredom or maybe created by it, but is not indicative of sleep debt. Nevertheless, sleepiness attracts much research effort, utilising tedious tests so sensitive to sleepiness; even a sleepiness not normally evident. The extent to which we are aware of our own sleepiness, without necessitating these tests, has medico-legal ramifications, even though it is argued, here, that this awareness is probably as good as these tests.

'Tiredness' is not synonymous with sleepiness, and although those with insomnia often attribute their tiredness to a lack of sleep, this is more of a feeling of weariness with a loss of interest in the world at large, which is distinct from sleepiness and a propensity to fall asleep. Such tiredness is not necessarily 'cured' by more sleep but, rather, by creating a better wakefulness. At the other extreme is the profound and perpetual sleepiness due to severe sleep disturbance seen with, for example, obstructive sleep apnoea syndrome, often unrecognised by sufferers, believing that they sleep well, but who remain perplexed as to why they are indeed so sleepy during the day.

Sleepiness is such a distinct aspect of sleep that it attracts considerable research attention, to the extent that other potentially important aspects of sleep are so easily overlooked. That is, sleep is not only for relieving sleepiness, inasmuch as eating food is not simply for relieving hunger, as the different nutrient contents of food have more subtle roles, as do the components of sleep, typically reflected by the EEG in the form of SWS and REM for example.

These less obvious roles of sleep takes *Sleeplessness* to the brain's cortex, especially its frontal region, comprising a third of our cortex, at its most highly developed in humans, and largely the seat of our uniquely human and subtle behaviours, collectively called 'executive functions', including those 'conscious decisions' of whether or not we decide to go to sleep. Until only a few decades ago this relatively huge brain region was thought to be 'surplus to requirements', mostly because there were no appropriate measures of such behaviours, all too easily missed under clinical and laboratory settings utilising relatively simple tests of brain function (an account of this historical oversight is given in the Appendix).

Today's research shows that even a single night of total sleep loss, as happens with long night shifts, causes temporary impairment to these executive functions, quickly reversed with recovery sleep. Such effects only really appear under real-world settings when we are confronted by unexpected, changing and challenging situations with competing distractions, requiring one to 'think out of the box', beyond routine responses; even when dealing with protracted, difficult overnight negotiations involving 'hidden agendas', and nuances in the behaviour of others. While caffeine and other 'psychostimulants' help overcome 'ordinary sleepiness', they have little benefit for these executive impairments.

SWS is also important for the ageing cortex in maintaining 'use it or lose it', in helping to create new connections during sleep that can help offset ageing effects. Although physical activity itself is thought to promote more of this cortical rewiring, there is more to this topic than at first seems, as the real benefit of such activity, especially for the frontal region, is not so much the exercise itself, but the extent to which it brings a variety of novel and interesting sensory and cognitive encounters with one's surroundings and people, to elicit new thoughts, emotions and experiences that need to be assimilated and remembered, leading to more SWS and its rewiring benefits. Whereas sitting reading or watching TV are too passive and less effective, all one really needs to 'exercise the cortex' are a comfortable pair of walking shoes, curiosity and a desire to explore.

So, here are some of the many topics to be covered in *Sleeplessness* in its critical appraisal of how much sleep we really need and what it is for, together with more reassuring perspectives on the beliefs concerning our apparent lack of sleep. Together, these might also provide further insights into insomnia, both for the individual and for that 'societal insomnia', otherwise seen as sleep debt.

Contents

List of Figures and Tables

Figures

Table

1

Insomnia

1.1   Sleeplessness: Lessons from History

Literature owes much to Charles Dickens' poor sleep when, on occasions, he would get out of bed and tramp the nighttime streets of London, encountering the people and places that gave him so many inspirations for his novels and for his conceptions of the tortured minds of many of his characters. His remarkable accounts of these wanderings and wonderings, which he called his 'houselessness', are described in his little known book of 'Night Walks', which might be seen as a positive side to insomnia and how he turned this affliction very much to his advantage. After walking for many miles, he would return home at sunrise, to his northwards pointing bed, to sleep exactly in the middle, placing his arms out and checking that his hands were equidistant from the bed's edge. At other times, when he could not sleep, he would stand at his bedside until feeling chilly, shake up and cool his pillows and bedclothes, then get back into bed. In fact, unlike the rest of his methods this latter technique is based on sound science as the body indeed needs to cool in order to ensure more rapid sleep onset.

© The Editor(s) (if applicable) and The Author(s) 2016
J. Horne, *Sleeplessness*, DOI 10.1007/978-3-319-30572-1_1

Nevertheless, his was a magnetic personality in more ways than one as, away from home, he would realign the bed to the north, which is why he always carried a compass—to foster his creativity as he also had to be facing north before he would put pen to paper. He believed in mesmerism (also called 'animal magnetism'), thought to be linked to real magnetism, as Mesmer, himself, would use pieces of magnetic iron ore ('lodestone') as part of his mesmeric treatments, even for curing insomnia. But this was too much for Dickens, who dismissed such use of magnets as 'unnatural'. Nevertheless, lodestones embedded in pillows were a very popular cure-all amongst the Victorians. But we shouldn't mock, as even in the 1960s, a 'magnetic field deficiency syndrome', with symptoms including insomnia, was a common diagnosis in Japan, and even today, magnetic pillows and mattresses continue to be advertised to alleviate insomnia.

However, Dickens, who died in 1870, couldn't really be called an 'insomniac' as the term was seldom used at the time. Yes, he suffered from insomnia, but then it was called 'sleeplessness', and another 30 or so years elapsed before 'insomnia' became the word of choice, coinciding with the development of new medicines and changes to medical practice (more about this, later).

Until then, the obvious remedies for sleeplessness were either alcohol (gin for the poor and whisky or brandy for the wealthier), or the readily accessible and cheaper 'fix' of opium in one form or another, with the most popular being laudanum, a tincture of alcohol and morphine. Being unrestricted, it could be bought almost anywhere. In fact, so popular was opium, that the British had largely gone to war with China, in the 'opium wars', to maintain the lucrative supplies. Byron, Shelley, de Quincey, Coleridge, Poe and even William Wilberforce were 'opium-eaters', using the drug not just as a sleeping aid, but also for pleasure or out of addiction. Meanwhile, cannabis, also easily available, was regarded to be more dangerous than laudanum, until it became known that Queen Victoria had been prescribed it by her personal physician, Dr JR Reynolds, to 'assist sleep during menstrual cramps'. Some years later, in 1890, he reflected in an article for the Lancet, that cannabis was 'one of the most valuable medicines we possess for treating insomnia'.

For those after a milder treatment for their sleeplessness, there was the herb valerian, named after the sleepless Roman emperor Publius Licinius Valerianus, who advocated its use throughout his empire. Although, pharmacologically, it had only a modest soporific effect, it benefited from having such an influential user and patron, and became the medicine of choice for the sleepless Romans, especially when coupled with the power of such a celebrity endorsement. Human nature being what it is, such placebo effects remain with us, more than ever with today's 'over-the-counter' remedies, including modern prescription medicines that are truly hypnotic, but also have additional placebo effects.

But to return to the Dickensian era, where there was good insight into insomnia, albeit quaintly amusing and still relevant today, lamentations about sleeplessness abounded in the then medical literature. For example, an editorial in the BMJ of 29 September 1894 (p. 279) bemoaned, "*The subject of sleeplessness is once more under public discussion. The hurry and excitement of modern life is held to be responsible for much of the insomnia of which we hear; and most of the articles and letters are full of good advice to live more quietly and of platitudes concerning the harmfulness of rush and worry. The pity of it is that so many people are unable to follow this good advice and are obliged to lead a life of anxiety and high tension*".

The editorial went on to review various attested treatments, pointing out that different remedies suit different people, to the extent that one apparently effective remedy can be the exact opposite of another. For example: hot baths versus cold baths, hot drinks versus cold drinks, long walks (in bare feet) versus sitting whilst attempting 'steady but monotonous counting' or 'the more difficult feat of thinking about nothing'. The article concluded with what must be the most extraordinary account of a cure, originally taken from the *Glasgow Herald*:

Soap your head with the ordinary yellow soap; rub it into the roots of the hair until your head is just lather all over, tie it up in a napkin, go to bed, and wash it out in the morning. Do this for a fortnight. Take no tea after 6 pm. I did this, and have never been troubled with sleeplessness since. I have lost sleep on an occasion since, but one or two nights of the soap cure put it right. I have conversed with medical men, but I have no explanation from any of them. All that I am careful about is that it cured me.

The editorial wisely ends with the comment that *"we cannot help thinking that some of our sleepless readers would prefer the disease to the cure. But if any should like to try it, may we advise that they should first, at any rate, follow that part of the advice which relates to the tea, and leave the soap part as a last resource"*.

The interesting word, here, was 'disease' , as this was still a time when 'the mind' was somewhat of a little understood, embarrassing enigma, largely ignored by physicians and well before the era of Freud and his contemporaries. None of the numerous remedies for sleeplessness involved anything along the lines of what one might call psychological therapy, even though stress and a troubled mind were well known to be the common basis, as reflected over 30 years earlier, in another insightful BMJ editorial (9 November 1861, p. 489), entitled 'On Sleeplessness', by Dr James Russell:

> *In treating these cases [of sleeplessness], the key to success lies in the management of the patient's mind, and unless we recognise the large share which is taken by mental disorder in producing and perpetuating the various and puzzling symptoms which present themselves, we shall not only fail in our object, but shall be in danger of actually aggravating the malady. Much may be done by soporifics and tonics; but our chief attention must be directed to regulating and strengthening the mind, otherwise our medicines will only serve to fix the patient's attention more closely upon the symptoms, and induce reliance upon external measures rather than upon self discipline. The treatment required is suggested by the nature of the malady. We find self-control diminished, the will inert, the emotions dominant, the thoughts of the sufferers occupied entirely about themselves, and the idea of disease the one subject engrossing their attention; we find every sensation registered, every fresh complaint welcomed and symptoms which at first seem to belong to organic disease are discovered, by further experience of the case, to have their origin in nothing but exaggerated sensitiveness or disordered fancy ... The task of ministering to such a condition is no light one; and it is hard to say whether the discipline is more severe to the patient or to the attendant ...*

This was also the era when fortitude and a 'stiff upper lip' were expected of patients, and when the prevailing medical opinion was that emotions caused bodily changes, particularly within the cardiovascular system, to the extent that treatments for 'emotional problems' often involved targeting the heart and blood in some way. It was certainly reflected by the Danish physician, Carl Lange, who claimed that, *"we owe all the emotional side of our mental life to our vasomotor system"*, which attracted much interest in Europe. He soon came to the attention of William James, the famous American philosopher and psychologist, who was thinking along similar lines, and invited Lange to co-author their renowned book, *The Emotions* (1887). Thus, the James–Lange theory of emotion was born, whereby emotions were the result of the perception of bodily changes. It also explains why insomnia, despite its link with stress and anxiety, continued to be viewed as a 'physical disorder' with so many treatments aimed at the heart one way or another, often with bizarre remedies. For example, the authoritative reference book on home management *The American Housekeeper's Encyclopedia* (1883), advocated, *"when overwakeful, get out of bed, dip a piece of cloth in water, lay this around the wrist; then wrap the dry portion over this and pin it, to keep it in place. This will exert a composing influence over the nervous system, and producing a sweet sleep, reducing the pulse; a handkerchief folded lengthwise will do. It is easy; try it."*

Absurd as this may be, the radial pulse in the wrist was seen as the primary medical route to the heart, and 'taking the pulse' was a comforting touch by the doctor for the patient. Thus many physicians saw sleeplessness as being due to insufficient blood flow somewhere in the body, often resulting in contrasting opinions. One school of thought believed that insomnia was due to brain congestion from excess blood in the head, reduced by being propped up by pillows. Another, that as there was insufficient blood in the brain, this was rectified by raising the feet, again with pillows. Of course, again, superstitious behaviour and the placebo effect were largely responsible for the efficacy of these treatments.

1.2 Insomnia: 'Medicalising' Sleeplessness?

By the 1890s a variety of new drugs had been discovered, and found to be effective in treating sleeplessness. Reinvigorated by this new armoury, the British Medical Association campaigned against what it called 'secret remedies' and forced the removal of opiates and cannabis (and also cocaine) from tonics and non-prescription medicines. Also, by now, physicians were responsible for prescribing most drugs, and the old style apothecaries had to cede to the professional pharmacists. Thus, medicine and its practice had become more powerful, especially as these new drugs provided real 'cures'. Moreover, sleeplessness, or insomnia as is was becoming known, was now increasingly attributed to 'brain dysfunction'—that is, still as a physical illness brought on by anxiety and stress but with little regard for tackling psychological cause. Given that physicians now had effective drug treatments, 'insomnia' as a diagnosis came into its own, and with its treatment solely under their control, this allowed the disorder to be medicalised to a much greater degree. Patients could be diagnosed as 'insomniacs' in their own right, rather than belittled for lacking moral fibre and becoming reliant on bizarre remedies or hopelessly addicted to opium.

Such a viewpoint was reflected by the distinguished John Buckley Bradbury, Professor of Medicine at Cambridge University, when he gave his influential Royal Society Lecture entitled, 'Some points connected with sleep, sleeplessness and hypnotics' (BMJ, 15 July 1899, p. 134). For him, "*the reason [for insomnia] is that the cerebral cells have assumed an irritable condition and it is necessary to depress their activity to bring them back to a more natural state ... it is here that hypnotics are of such great value*". Paraldehyde, chloralamide, chloralose, chloral hydrate, sulphonal, potassium bromide were seen to be the least harmful ...' He also recommended "*a scantily furnished, quiet, well ventilated bedroom, having moderate temperature, with light excluded, and that there be a firm mattress, light, warm bedding*". Despite many pages in each of four successive issues of the BMJ being devoted to his further lectures on sleeplessness, he made little mention of anything which could be interpreted as psychological treatment of the underlying causes, apart from remarks such as: "*sleeplessness from overwork especially literary work requires mental rest and change of air and scene*". As well as: "*cool air of bedroom, wet pack, whisky and water ... Hang feet out of bed, walk about naked, rub feet if cold ...*" Nevertheless he did note that the treatment of insomnia was "*one of the most difficult subjects in therapeutics ... have a number of drugs ... given in sufficient doses ... produce a desired result ... may make the patient a slave to the habit ... more disasterous than the insomnia itself*" (p. 136).

More hypnotics appeared with such rapidity that it was impossible to compare their advantages and disadvantages as sleep producers. In the cool light of day, so to speak, it soon became apparent that all these hypnotics had greater side effects than anticipated, and were often too slow in producing sleep at night, which in turn was too prolonged, with subsequent sleepiness lasting well into the next day, and with giddiness and incoordination. Worse still, the same hypnotic would have worryingly different effects between patients.

Cautious, supposedly more insightful, articles soon appeared in the BMJ, notably in another series of reported lectures, in 1900 (beginning 1 December, pp. 551–553), and entitled 'Causes and Cure of Insomnia', by the eminent physician Sir James Sawyer. For him, insomnia was not so much a problem for the working classes, as it was associated with mental not physical work, as it (insomnia) *"occurs mostly in persons who are members of what are known as the upper and middle classes … mostly in persons of high mental endowment and of neurotic temperament"*. Unlike the working class patient, who probably never saw a doctor anyway, as they could not afford his fees, Sir James went on to note that *"Work which prevents due sleep is dangerous work. When a man cannot sleep because he works his brain too much, we make as a condition of our help that he stop or greatly lessen his labour; especially should he abstain from mental work for some hours before going to bed … Be wisely suspicious as to accepting work as a cause of insomnia … It is mostly worry, not overwork, or it is work under wrong conditions which brings unrest."*

Mindful of rather wealthy patients with much time to spare, he advocated holidays with a complete change of scene, *and "the present therapeutic worship of the sun, and you will find free and long daily exposure to sunshine a valuable adjuvant in the cure of insomnia"*. However, we now know how important daylight or artificial light is in stabilising the body clock (see Sect. 8.2), coupled with his *"get up at fixed and regular times … healthy sleep is a rhythmic act"*.

More of his wiser words came with *"Give hypnotics only in exceptional cases; only administer such drugs when you cannot help it"*. However, he did recommend a *"nightcap of toddy (alcohol) … which should be discontinued when the conditions which called for it shall have disappeared"*.

Today we hear of 'mindfulness', a contemporary term adopted to describe a meditational state largely originating from Sanskrit and early Buddhism, whereby one focuses attention on an emotion or body sensation, usually breathing, thus helping to clear the mind. Remarkably, Sir James also suggested a similar technique for insomnia, with the sufferer lying on their right side, in bed, head on a pillow, and taking "*full inspiration … as much as possible through the nostrils … such that respiration neither to be accelerated not retarded too much … with breath passing through the nostrils in a continuous stream*". Such breathing in and out continues so that, "*the mind is to conceive this apart from all other ideas apart from and breathing*" until the "*hypnotic faculty steeps it in oblivion*". Which is almost exactly the same as is recommended by psychologists today.

Sadly, few of today's practitioners have ever heard of Sir James Sawyer or his contemporaries, but we need to be reminded that so much of what is known today about insomnia has been said before, albeit rather more eloquently and using less prosaic terminology than is found in the statements used today.

1.3   Today

Life doesn't really change, and neither has our insight into insomnia, regardless of much new research that has provided more refined diagnoses and treatments. Around half of those people with insomnia suffer from 'primary' insomnia [1] as, ostensibly, there is no 'medical or psychiatric cause', or other sleep disorder (e.g. 'periodic leg movements in sleep'—see Sect. 9.4), or substance or alcohol abuse. Despite having every opportunity in obtaining good sleep these sufferers have difficulty in going to sleep, staying asleep, maybe waking up too early and, overall, see their sleep to be of too poor a quality, often leaving them unable to concentrate, and being forgetful and moody during the day. Whilst in bed trying (often too hard) to sleep there are frequent intrusive and persistent racing thoughts, leaving one tense and unable to relax. Needless to say, this leads to daytime worries and more ruminations about sleep, to the point that it can become the focus of waking life, together with the tendency to complain of being 'tired all the time'. Often, sleep is better away from home, where many of those unwanted associations are left behind.

In contrast, other forms of insomnia, usually referred to as 'secondary' or 'comorbid' insomnia [1] have more obvious physical causes such as pain, neurological and cardiovascular disorders, as well as psychiatric problems, or more external causes such as noise and shift work. Clearly, treatment, here, has to try and deal with those more specific causes. Of course, there might well be an understandable anxiety and emotional component to these causes as well, hence the term 'comorbid'.

In *Sleeplessness* I will be concentrating on primary insomnia, with it being the most common form of insomnia suffered by many people, which often has stress and anxiety as its basis. Clinicians also refer to primary insomnia as 'psychophysiological insomnia' [1], as the anxiety heightens various body functions, most noticeably heart rate and general metabolism which, together, cause a persistent and underlying agitation and a feeling of being unable to unwind and relax throughout the day and night, and hence there is a persistent state of 'hyperarousal' [1]. **Throughout the rest of this book I will be referring to this primary insomnia, just as 'insomnia',** which those Victorians mostly saw as 'sleeplessness'.

1.4 Severity

Insomnia is one of the few disorders that a physician will usually let their patient self-diagnose without any real examination, at least during initial consultations, and then usually offer a prescription for hypnotics. Such an expediency by a time-pressed physician is understandable in the short term. Nevertheless, it is difficult for the doctor to determine the severity of the insomnia and various assessment questionnaires have been developed either for the patient to complete or doctor to ask. Let me briefly describe the one [2] developed by Dr Charles Morin and his group from the University of Laval, in Quebec, whose questionnaire is based on their extensive studies of people with insomnia. It is succinct in having just seven items identifying the nature, severity and impact of insomnia. Responses are on a five-point scale, from 'no problem' (=0) to 'very severe problem' (=4), with the patient having to 'think back for the previous month', and 'rate yourself (0–4) on the following':

1. Severity of getting to sleep;
2. Maintaining sleep;
3. Early morning awakening;
4. Sleep dissatisfaction;
5. Interference of sleep difficulties with daytime functioning;
6. Noticeability of sleep problem by others;
7. Patient distress due to the sleep difficulties.

The scores are totalled and the patient is classified as:
Having no problem with insomnia 0–7;
'Sub-threshold' insomnia 8–14;
Moderate insomnia 15–21;
Severe insomnia 22–28.

The physician then decides whether and how to treat the insomnia, depending on its severity.

All seven of these categories are seen to be of equal importance. Notably, the last four items (4–7) deal with the perceived consequences of the first three, with the patient's concern about these consequences often being worse than the symptoms themselves. For the first four, the greatest problem for patients is usually not with falling asleep, but with question 2, staying asleep, followed by question 3, early morning awakening. Nevertheless, much of today's research into drug treatment has tended to be in dealing with the first question, in falling asleep. Moreover, the underlying anxiety, hyperarousal, and the patient's other worries about what will happen to mind and body with insufficient sleep are often overlooked during short consultations, ending with that prescription for a hypnotic. This is why psychological therapies dealing with the mind are so important, as they place the control of the underlying causes and treatment into the patient's hands, rather than just relying on hypnotics, which are still useful in the short term but should be used in conjunction with the longer-term benefits of psychological methods.

Given these different levels of severity of insomnia, it can be seen how estimates about the prevalence of insomnia in a population can vary quite considerably, depending on how it is defined and its frequency, as many surveys merely just refer to 'insomnia' or 'poor sleep' in very general terms. Moreover, whereas insomnia seems to be more frequent in women than men, this may be at least in part due to denial by men, whereas women are generally more forthcoming about their health problems.

One of the main purposes of *Sleeplessness* is to allay fears about the consequences of inadequate sleep in those suffering from insomnia, by looking at the scientific and medical evidence behind various findings and adverse claims, which are often embellished by the media, only to further add to the anxieties of sufferers, and hence worsen their condition.

1.5 Contradictions

Although there have been claims that insomnia might have a marked 'inherited' aspect, this has yet to be established, as there are many instances of family histories of insomnia largely due to traditional family behaviours and practices, passed down the generations, and is not so 'genetic' as might first seem. Apart from any apparent genetic inheritability being likely to depend on numerous genes, one has also to consider whether there is some other behavioural characteristic that has been overlooked, but also reflected by insomnia. Thus when trying to determine some hereditary aspect to any behaviour, including insomnia, it is necessary to look at relatives living under different physical, social and emotional environments, and note the extent to which the behaviour remains. Besides, the impact of many of the genes affecting behaviour can be modified or suppressed by various environments and other external pressures, through a process called 'epigenetics' whereby genes are naturally switched on or off due to external and environmental factors.

Some researchers have created 'models of insomnia' by giving laboratory rodents lesions to brain areas that seem to create insomnia in these animals, in an attempt to understand the brain mechanisms underlying insomnia, even the effectiveness of hypnotics. However, it is difficult to see how this approach can be reconciled with the psychological 'state of mind' in human sufferers. This is rather like assuming that as heart rate is higher in people with insomnia, largely due to their hyperarousal, then an animal model would be to interfere with the mechanisms directly controlling heart rate, causing it to increase. But this would largely bypass an underlying cause, anxiety. Another model of insomnia has utilised caffeine given to healthy human volunteers to create artificial hyperarousal and thus impaired sleep. Again, though, this is not comparable with real insomnia as, for example, patients also focus on the consequences of their insomnia, whereas this is not usually the case with 'caffeinated normals'.

There is no evidence of brain damage or lesions in those people with insomnia, although there may be reversible reductions to blood flow to certain brain areas in long-term sufferers, especially within the frontal area of cortex; even when it is smaller in size, in some cases [3]. This highly developed human brain area (see Chap. 10) which, by the way, is poorly developed in rodents, is involved with our ability to deal with more complex decisions, assimilating new experiences, avoiding distractions and multitasking, for example. Thus, these reductions in blood flow may well be linked to the chronic hyperarousal, with such sufferers tending to focus their waking thoughts and actions more 'inwardly' than on the ongoing outside world, to the extent that they make lesser use of this brain area. However, this should not be of too great a concern as our cortex is highly 'plastic' (unlike that of the rodent) and adapts with use. So this effect is likely to reverse after a few months when the insomnia has been resolved and when the sufferer has re-engaged more fully with the world at large.

1.6   Ambiguities

An apparent paradox, often seen with people with insomnia attending a sleep clinic, is a considerable difference between the duration of sleep monitored overnight by an EEG and other measures, known as 'polysomnography' (PSG) [4], compared with what the patient reports. For example, there can be up to a threefold difference between what is measured and what the patient states as the time it took them to fall asleep, with the patient often quite certain about their longer estimate. This 'sleep state misperception' [1] as it is called, has a plausible explanation linked to the hyperarousal. When we begin to fall asleep, in bed with eyes shut, the transition from wake to sleep becomes blurred to the point that it is difficult to know whether one is asleep or awake, as the sense of time is quite distorted. The process of falling asleep for all of us, good or bad sleepers, is not sudden, and usually begins with drifting in and out of what can be quite good sleep, for the first 10 minutes or thereabouts after lights out, interspersed with maybe around 5 seconds or so of wakefulness when the normal sleeper will typically change positions to become more comfortable. Whereas the normal sleeper will need only a few minutes of this initial sleep in order to know that they have drifted off to sleep, those with insomnia need around 15–20 minutes of sustained sleep before they know this. Instead, they perceive these longer periods of drifting in and out of sleep as persistent wakefulness.

Moreover, many people with insomnia usually do not have any marked sleep loss when their sleep is assessed by PSG [3], and neither is there any obvious degree of daytime sleepiness, which should otherwise be evident. Although one might simply argue that the hyperarousal counteracts or hides any sleepiness caused by lost sleep, there is little evidence of this, as will be seen. Yet, there are often feelings of 'unrefreshing sleep' and being 'tired all the time', pointing to what the patient and their own doctor may believe to be sleepiness, but this tiredness is often something different (see Sect. 1.13).

Moreover, when asked to complete the Epworth Sleepiness Scale (ESS) [5], which determines one's general level of daytime sleepiness, those with insomnia usually report normal alertness. The ESS, which is described more fully in Sect. 9.2, requires people to think back over the previous few weeks, and respond to questions asking about the likelihoods of their actually dozing off under various unstimulating everyday situations, such as when watching TV, sitting as a passenger in a car, quietly reading, etc. The scale is quite different from the other subjective sleepiness scales I'll be coming to in Sect. 8.4, assessing sleepiness as it is presently felt.

A more objective measure of sleepiness often used in the sleep clinic, which also fails to show much by way of sleepiness in patients with insomnia, is the Multiple Sleep Latency Test (MSLT). Here, the patient lies on a comfortable bed in a darkened room, with their EEG monitored to record the onset of any sleep. They are asked to 'relax and try to go to sleep'. The test lasts for 20 minutes and is usually repeated four times, every two hours, typically from 10 a.m. As soon as 15 seconds of sleep are detected the session is ended, as any longer sleep might well interfere with potential sleepiness in the next session. The rationale is that the faster the onset of sleep, the greater is the sleepiness, with the average time taken to do this over all the sessions being the 'MSLT score'. If the patient does not fall sleep in the time available, the score is given as 20 minutes.

Suffice to say that, mostly, these patients usually do not fall asleep more quickly than the norm. Of course, it could be argued that such a test is pointless, given that sufferers have difficulties in falling asleep at night, anyway, which could carry over into the test itself. On the other hand, other sensitive measures of sleepiness, especially tedious psychological performance tests, such as 'simple reaction time' tests, also tend not to show any impairment [6]. Again, it could be the 'hyperarousal' masking or otherwise counteracting any increased propensity to be sleepy during the test. Of course, patients attending clinics, especially for the measurement of MSLTs can be apprehensive, as one might well be in attending a clinic of any sort, which may only add to their hyperarousal. This might be further enhanced by various activities and concerns on route to the clinic. If patients are not given adequate assurances and plenty of time to settle down before the MSLT, then this only adds to the further potential pointlessness of the test.

Many with insomnia complain that they cannot concentrate at work, which could indeed indicate excess sleepiness, especially as there are clear findings showing that some, but more complex, psychological performance tests do indicate impairment [7]. Although this poor concentration may be a consequence of underlying worries, with persistent ruminations about the insomnia, there is another explanation here, unrelated to sleepiness, due to the hyperarousal, as I will now describe.

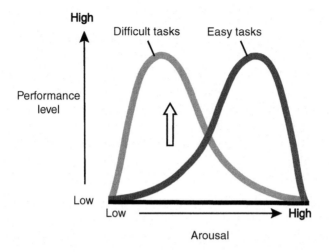

Fig. 1.1 Optimum performance differs between easy and difficult tasks according to arousal level

1.7 'Inverted U'

It is well known in psychology, that whilst arousal or anxiety will increase one's performance at simple tasks up to a point, in contrast, it leads to a deterioration in more complex and demanding ones. This association between arousal and performance is known as the 'inverted U' and is seen in Fig. 1.1, whereby there is an optimal level of arousal for tasks differing in complexity. It can be seen that for an easy task, such as tedious and simple reaction time tests, an increased arousal level, as with hyperarousal, and shown by the arrow, leads to performance improvement up to a point, thereafter falling as arousal becomes very high. On the other hand, for more demanding and difficult tasks, optimal performance is at a much lower threshold on the arousal scale (as shown by the vertical arrow). Thus for patients with hyperarousal, they still may be somewhat under the optimum 'hill' with easy tasks, able to do even better perhaps, but are well over the hill for difficult ones [7]. When patients are successfully treated for hyperarousal, normal performance returns, inasmuch as there is a shift to the left on the arousal curve. Thus they tend to become slower on the simple tasks and better on the complex ones [7], all of which might explain why those with insomnia can have difficulties in the workplace when the job is likely to comprise relatively complex tasks, as well as cause 'presenteeism' (see Sect. 1.12).

Difficult tasks also involve driving, not so much on motorways and other monotonous roads when driving is more routine and comparable with simpler performance tasks, but in towns when driving is more demanding. Thus, applying the 'inverted U' and with hyperarousal, sufferers are unlikely to have accidents (or fall asleep at the wheel) during undemanding motorway driving, as they are still on the ascendant of that U, but are more likely to have a 'prang' with demanding urban driving, as their performance here is 'over the hill' and on the decline.

1.8   Lack of Sleep?

If and when someone with insomnia is referred to a sleep clinic and undergoes overnight assessment by PSG, to eliminate more serious sleep disorders, it is unlikely that this will add much more insight into the insomnia, apart from identifying 'sleep state misperception', mentioned earlier. In fact, in most cases, their total sleep time as actually measured, here, is typically within normal limits for their age and gender, despite their maybe spending somewhat longer in getting to sleep as, nevertheless, sleep usually lasts at least 6 hours [4]. Similarly, the quality of this sleep is usually not as bad as the patient might believe, and is often within normal limits, despite some greater degree of waking up after sleep onset [1]. On the other hand, it might be countered that these patients are inherently longer sleepers than healthy controls, such that the 6 hours' sleep they obtain is indeed too short. In which case maybe they do suffer from chronically insufficient sleep?

However, for many sufferers, sleeping away from home and all its emotional associations helps them to relax more at bedtime, and thus allow for better sleep. One is reminded of the old adage that 'a change is as good as a rest' (even though the hyperarousal remains [8]). This outcome is even apparent when sleeping in the clinic, involving a sense of a patient's relief with the thought that 'something will now be done about my insomnia'. But the effect varies, as other patients remain apprehensive and continue to underestimate their total sleep in the clinic, to a greater extent than when at home.

Nevertheless, apart from these issues, people with insomnia should not add to their worries in believing that they are not obtaining that '8 hours a night', which is still commonly but mistakenly advocated by the media, and often by friends and family alike. Similarly unfounded are any further worries that their apparent lack of 8 hours' sleep will lead to cardiovascular disease and obesity, which are the topics of Chaps. 3 and 4. Such worries only further increase stress and the levels of the stress coping hormone, cortisol [9], often seen with chronic insomnia, and linked to the hyperarousal [1, 10].

Few studies have really targeted the hyperarousal, in trying to reduce it rather than aim at the perceived poor sleep. Work by pioneering researchers in this field of insomnia, Drs Mike Bonnet and Donna Anand [9, 11] at the VA hospital in Dayton, Ohio, offers some degree of hope by concentrating on and reducing this hyperarousal. They find that exercise regimens aiming to improve physical fitness, with reductions both in resting metabolic rate and in measures of stress, lead to sleep improvement, at least in the short term. But whether this can be maintained in the long term remains a debatable point, as long-term exercise studies, lasting for a year, find only marginally significant trends for sleep improvement (in older women, e.g. [12]), although this is greater for those whose physical fitness has improved the best [12].

1.9 Sleeping Tablets

Extending or otherwise improving sleep at night with modern-day hypnotics is unlikely to increase alertness the next day [1] for those with insomnia, largely because they are already quite alert anyway, from the hyperarousal. Yet they may feel better having felt more reassured about their sleep. Although sleeping tablets are useful as part of the initial treatment for insomnia, these are only a partial solution. After a few weeks of taking any nightly tablet, whatever it is, few people with insomnia will actually have their sleep increased by more than 30 minutes, which is largely due to a similar reduction in the time they take to fall asleep, as measured by PSG. Nevertheless, many of these medicines also help by acting as tranquillisers, by reducing anxiety and worries at bedtime, to improve relaxation while lying there waiting to get to sleep, and perhaps leading to greater satisfaction the next day. To the extent that this waking contentment might help alleviate hyperarousal, there will then be some improvement to those more demanding complex tests I mentioned, involving that 'inverted U'.

Arguably, half the benefit from any modern sleeping tablet or other preparation, be it prescribed or just bought over the counter, is due to what the patient will believe will happen; that is, the placebo effect. Confidence in any treatment acts as a powerful therapeutic tool, as it might be in buying that new mattress. This is because the real secret of conquering insomnia is peace of mind at bedtime. In a study we undertook with volunteer poor sleepers, looking at the placebo effect in a harmless way, we utilised a bedtime drink well known through its advertising and impressive packaging and advice on better sleep. Our other condition comprised the identical drink but packaged in a plain plastic pot, with the participants told that this was a new drink about to come on the market, and we had no idea as to its effectiveness in helping sleep. In contrast we said that the other, in its usual package, was believed to be quite effective.

Thus, what differed between the drinks was the packaging and our short comment about the product. Participants tried both samples, for a week at a time, in a 'crossover design' whereby half the participants tried one sample before the other, and the other half, the reverse order. All kept 'sleep diaries' logging each morning how long it took them to fall asleep, for how long they slept, and how they felt on awakening next morning. All reported that the attractively presented version was superior in all these respects, especially in reducing the time to get to sleep by up to a perceived half an hour. This outcome is not to decry the 'real' product as it does work, especially as it is both inexpensive in terms of dose and is harmless, all of which I applaud. Of course, this was a fairly crude study, but it again points to the powerful effect of 'mind over matter' which, in terms of the placebo effect, has yet to be fully addressed even in the newer hypnotics, of which there are many.

Given the usual shortage of the consultation period for when people see their doctor, physicians are unable to talk through underlying anxieties and waking pressures that might underlie the insomnia. On the other hand, practitioners of alternative therapies will usually devote a much longer time in listening sympathetically and impartially to their client, often for a much longer duration than the client has ever experienced before, and when providing the therapy itself. Hence, the whole experience is likely to be of far greater benefit than the actual therapy alone. So, for example, if the therapy involves a pleasant aroma from oils or whatever, to be utilised at bedtime, then the benefits to sleep might not so much be from this substance itself, but from recalling the entire therapeutic milieu, stimulated by the aroma or whatever, and thus quite comforting.

Most sleeping tablets are 'short-acting' in lasting only for a few hours and aimed at speeding up sleep onset, whereas Morin's findings [2], mentioned earlier, showed that more distressing for those with insomnia was waking up a few hours after sleep onset and then being unable to return to sleep for what might seem to be an interminable time. To treat the latter, a longer acting hypnotic would be needed, lasting well into this wake-up zone. But then there is the risk that this effect lasts too long, leading to daytime grogginess. In fact the design of the perfect hypnotic largely remains beyond our reach, at least so far. Ideally it should have all the following properties that mostly come under the heading of 'pharmacokinetics': it is quickly absorbed from the stomach into the blood and thence into the brain (thus having to be taken almost while getting into bed), to rapidly induce a natural sleep that is prolonged for, say, 6 hours, at which point it has largely been eliminated from the body, to leave a natural waking up without hangover effects and, instead, a feeling of well-being the next day.

It must be safe in overdose, without any side effects such as: interfering with balance when walking to the toilet at night, or with breathing during sleep, or interactions with other drugs including alcohol (despite patients being told to avoid alcohol at bedtime), is able to be taken every night without any deterioration in effect (i.e. no 'tolerance' and thus no need to keep increasing the dose), and no rebound insomnia or withdrawal effects when it is stopped being taken. A near-impossible task for such a wonder drug, of course, as would be the cost of developing it. And then there is the problem of marked differences between people in the effectiveness of most, if not all, hypnotics as, like most medicines, there is no universal panacea in providing all things to all people.

Nevertheless, hypnotics can be tailored to individual requirements, at least to some extent as, for example, there are those that are designed to induce sleep fairly quickly and then soon disappear from the body, compared with those that last for much of the night, or are have a delayed release in only acting a few hours into sleep, to offset unwanted mid-sleep awakenings. The technical term relating to all this, is 'plasma elimination half-life' or just 'half-life'. This is the time taken for 50 % of the drug to be eliminated from the blood (but not necessarily from the body), and thus it is assumed to be much less effective at that point, although in some cases the breakdown products of the drug, still remaining in the blood, can also have a soporific effect, despite the drug itself having largely disappeared. This happened with some older sleeping tablets that appeared to have short half-lives, but with less desirable breakdown products that produced waking hangover effects. Such complications also vary between people, depending on individual differences in one's body biochemistry, particularly in the liver and kidneys, where most of the drug disposal takes place. This is a problem most evident with the elderly where there is a natural decline in the ability of the ageing kidney and liver to dispose of these and other medicines, to the extent that the unwanted carry-over effect into the daytime can be marked. Thus, getting the dose just right can be very difficult with the elderly, and sometimes almost impossible if other medications are involved.

Many elderly usually have little difficulty in falling asleep at night, but become distressed with too early a morning awakening. For them the design of a hypnotic that is effective in delaying this awakening, without causing oversleep and daytime grogginess, still remains problematic, although the hormone melatonin, which I will be describing in more detail in Sect. 7.1, is sometimes useful here, given as a tablet taken an hour or so before sleep at night. Although not really a hypnotic, but a natural hormone, it is rather slow in acting, unlike true hypnotics, but helps to realign the circadian body clock and boosts the positioning of nighttime sleep, especially in older adults and the elderly where this clock has weakened. Such a melatonin boost at night not only provides for better sleep timing and quality, but can delay that early morning awakening. As far as it is known, melatonin has no hangover effects. However, because daylight and bright indoor light naturally increase alertness and counteract the effects of melatonin, the two should not be used at the same time, but alternately over the 24-hour period; that is, daylight and bright indoor light throughout the day and into the early evening, followed by the melatonin tablet. Moreover, bright light by day reduces daytime napping (often taken to excess in the elderly) and thus encourages more sleep at night.

For younger people, too short an acting hypnotic that disappears too rapidly (i.e. a short half-life) can just lead to a rebound insomnia a few hours later which, in effect, just shifts the insomnia from the beginning of sleep to mid-sleep. This is what an excess of evening alcohol intake tends to do. It certainly induces sleep, or rather, more of a torpor, as well as heavy snoring (Sect. 9.3), but as alcohol has this short half-life (depending on the dose and the individual), it disappears from the blood fairly rapidly, leaving this relatively sudden alcohol withdrawal to cause an agitated awakening a few hours into sleep. In fact, alcohol is a good example of how 'half-life' can be misleading in terms of effects on behaviour, as blood alcohol levels may well have returned to near zero by the morning, but there can be residual effects as felt with that hangover.

The extent to which sleeping tablets maintain their effect with repeated use, without necessitating having to increase the dose because one has developed 'tolerance' to the drug, remains a matter for debate, despite claims that this is unlikely with modern drugs. No present day sleeping tablet is addictive, as was found with the no longer prescribed barbiturates, for example. But people, today, can still become psychologically overdependent on them, especially in the longer term, and become agitated and overconcerned about a worsening of insomnia on stopping their medication; thus they return to taking the tablet. What often happens is that, as soon as one ceases taking one's usual tablet for just a night, this can result in poorer sleep for both psychological and pharmacological reasons. Because the insomnia seems to have returned with vengeance, then to avoid it happening the following night, the sleeping tablet is again resorted to, with sleep seeming to be much improved. However, because a better night's sleep would probably have happened anyway, as a good night usually naturally follows a bad one, too much of that sleep improvement is attributed to the tablet, and thus reinforces the need to continue with the nightly hypnotic.

A more reassuring method of withdrawing from sleeping tablets is, gradually over successive nights, to tailor the dose down until nothing is used, and then just take the tablet if it is ever needed. Having it resting on the bedside table gathering dust, and knowing it's there, just in case, can be therapeutic in itself. Which might be just as good as actually swallowing it, although this is not of much consolation for the pharmaceutical companies. Here, cognitive behaviour therapy (see next section) is particularly effective in handling this withdrawal. In fact, evidence is sparse that improved sleep from using sleeping tablets alone, leads to meaningful improvements in daytime well-being [13], or even with work performance [14], which again suggest that insomnia is more likely to be the result of poor well-being and quality of life, rather than vice versa.

Two final points. Although nowadays most doctors will only provide new prescriptions for hypnotics for one to two weeks of treatment, in the hope that the insomnia is only temporary, nevertheless, most prescriptions are renewals, and repeated for months, even years. Yet it is important that both doctor and patient can agree on an 'exit strategy' for dealing with ceasing the hypnotic, although many patients will then resort to less effective, albeit harmless but expensive over-the-counter sleep aids. Secondly, there are many medicines and other treatments for insomnia producing improvements to sleep, which have been shown to be statistically significantly better than a placebo when given 'double-blind'; that is neither the patient nor the investigator knows which is which. The assumption is then generally made that this level of improvement is also clinically significant and of real benefit to the patient, which well it may be. However, sometimes these former improvements may only be small and only evident if the sample size is relatively large, and thus only really providing changes of clinically marginal improvement. This issue of statistical versus clinical significance is of considerable importance to many areas of medicine, and it is all too easy to assume that these terms are synonymous. I will be raising this point again in Sect. 3.2 in another sleep-related context.

1.10 Cognitive Behaviour Therapy for Insomnia (CBT-i)

Insomnia is often long lasting, with its more enduring treatments requiring professional counselling, enabling the patient to understand and deal with their waking worries beyond the insomnia. This is important, as simply focusing on the sleep alone, near bedtime, is unlikely to markedly improve one's quality of life to any real extent. This is why the more specialised cognitive behaviour therapy for insomnia (CBT-i) can be so effective. This psychological technique targets the various underlying causes of insomnia, especially sleep-related anxieties and sleep-interfering behaviours, as well as the often disorganised sleep itself. Apart from CBT-i usually being able to deal with these worries and stresses of waking life that may well have caused the insomnia in the first place, there is also a series of techniques known as 'stimulus controls', designed first to undo those well-engrained negative associations with persistent unsuccessful attempts to sleep, and then to substitute more appropriate behaviours, which, in effect, are designed to associate the bed with good sleep and pleasurable activities rather than be a site of misery and ordeal.

Stimulus controls include the following advice:

1. Only go to bed when feeling sleepy, irrespective of the time.
2. Abandon the bed if unable to sleep within, say, 20 minutes, and do something distracting in another room, not associated with sleep. This helps block out ruminating thoughts that would otherwise persist whilst lying awake in bed. Only return to bed when sleepiness appears and repeat as necessary. Lying awake at night struggling to get to sleep is pointless. But what to do? Passively reading or watching TV is often not effective, as one's mind just goes back to those worrying thoughts, with nothing read or watched being absorbed. People try various relaxation exercises and listen to recorded sounds, for example, of the sea or of birds. I favour doing a modest-sized jigsaw (not under bright light), which is relaxing and absorbing, thus helping to distract one from those worrying thoughts, especially when searching and sorting through those pieces. The physical activity of moving one's hands

about in doing this further adds to the distraction. When the eyes eventually become heavy with sleepiness, then it's time to return to bed. Besides, unlike some other sleep aids, jigsaws are cheap to buy especially from charity shops and can easily be swapped.

3. Some people find that a quiet, nighttime walk, maybe with the dog, is particularly relaxing and 'helps clear the mind', with sleep the better for doing this.

4. Avoid 'clock watching'. Set the morning alarm and then put the clock out of sight.

5. Avoid bright light and staring at a bright computer or tablet screen before bed as these have an alerting effect (see Sect. 7.1), as can further anxieties caused by 'must check my emails and texts before I go to sleep'.

6. Take comfort in knowing that if sleep is particularly bad that night, a better sleep will likely follow the next night, due to the sleep deprivation.

7. No matter what sleep was like that night, always arise at the same time each morning and, as soon as possible, get plenty of bright light whether it be indoors or daylight, as this helps re-establish the timing of sleep within the circadian body clock, as insomnia often desynchronises these two processes (see Sect. 6.2).

8. Limit daytime naps to around 15 minutes, otherwise, sleep pressure at night will be weakened.

These and other straightforward methods, advocated by CBT-i, substituting good for bad associations, can be easier said than done, and may take a few weeks fully to set in. Hence it is likely that they will cause some sleep deprivation, with daytime sleepiness, which can be off-putting, but perseverance is generally rewarding.

An additional technique is sleep restriction, whereby only about a 5-hour window of 'sleep opportunity' at night is allowed initially, which increases sleep pressure, and is aimed at improving sleep quality by gradually compressing interim waking periods during sleep. As the same morning wake-up time has to be maintained, this procedure entails a later bedtime, and a greater sleepiness, then. Although increased daytime sleepiness is likely for a while, it reinforces one's confidence in achieving a better sleep. With sleep quality improved by this rather procrustean approach, the sleep period can then be lengthened by, say, half-hourly amounts every few days, by bringing forwards the bedtime. As anxiety about sleep should also begin to diminish, so should the hyperarousal. Although successful treatment may not result in sleep extending beyond 6 hours (which is usually sufficient—see Chap. 6), even after a further 6 months' follow-up [15] patients are happier in themselves, even though some noticeable interim wakefulness during night sleep may remain, albeit usually noticeably reduced.

The various components of CBT-i provide for an effective treatment of insomnia, able to produce worthwhile and enduring results in a relatively brief number of reassuring visits to the therapist. Systematic reviews of CBT-i indicate that it has greater effectiveness than sleeping tablets, especially beyond six months or so after therapy is completed [16], even though around 30 % of sufferers tend to relapse into their old ways.

Finally, many people with insomnia keep detailed sleep diaries, before, during and after treatments, noting after each night when and how they slept. Some sleep specialists encourage this, so that progress becomes more evident, but this method can simply focus on the insomnia rather than on the real underlying waking problems. Besides, those bad nights of sleep, often meticulously recorded in the diary, sometimes with personal, lamentable feelings at the time, ought to be forgotten, not written down and kept as a constant reminder of times past. People can become quite irrational and superstitious about their sleep diaries, believing that if they don't make a complete entry for each night, sleep will get worse, so further adding to their concerns. Disposing of the diary, even ritualistically, and certainly at the beginning of any therapy, should be seen to portend the era of better sleep.

1.11 Sleep Hygiene

This is a rather unfortunately named collective term commonly used, mostly in the media, to describe well-meaning advice given to people with insomnia. At face value it suggests that insomnia is improved by clean bed linen and plenty of fresh air in the bedroom. Nevertheless, the advice tends to be rather strict with various 'don'ts', with the patient having to endure some suffering rather than comfort at bedtime, that can only add to the anxieties and woes of the poor sleeper. I'm reminded of the saying 'a little of what you fancy does you good', which seemingly contradicts several of the prescriptions of 'sleep hygiene'. For example, one is urged to, 'avoid alcohol at bedtime', which contrasts with the potential relaxing value of a 'small nightcap' maybe added to warm milk. Of course, consuming much more than this amount of alcohol, in an attempt to create oblivion, will markedly interfere with sleep, apart from the rebound agitation a few hours into sleep, as I explained earlier. Excess alcohol causes or worsens heavy snoring and obstructive sleep apnoea (Sect. 9.3), including more nocturnal trips to the toilet.

'Keep the bedroom darkened' is another such recommendation which might prevent reading an enjoyable and relaxing good book in bed. Another, to 'avoid caffeine', which does make sense, often includes chocolate, even though this usually contains only nominal amounts of caffeine, and thus might spoil the delight that chocolate in one form or another can give us in the evening. Interestingly, homeopathic treatments for insomnia, utilising the maxim of treating 'like with like' but in much diluted forms, utilise caffeine but in miniscule amounts. Lastly, advocating 'no daytime napping' can be taken to extremes in assuming this to be detrimental to nighttime sleep, whereas this is unlikely to apply to very short (15 minute) naps that can be so relaxing and unwinding.

Then there is the belief in the need to strive for at least 7 hours' or maybe 8 hours' sleep, seemingly required to avoid the apparent scourge of 'sleep debt', which I will be covering in the next few chapters.

Waking up feeling 'unrefreshed', often taken as a sign of poor sleep, which well it might be, is a term widely used in assessing sleep quality and quantity, but given its vagueness it is so liable to misinterpretation. Besides, many good sleepers require several minutes after waking up in the morning before becoming fully 'refreshed', as the transition from sleep is not instantaneous, and neither is the process of falling asleep at night, which can also take several minutes. Feeling refreshed on awakening also relates to one's degree of morningness–eveningness (Sect. 7.3), as 'owls', unlike 'larks' take longer to come round after waking up in the morning, which is not necessarily a sign of poor sleep.

1.12 Overwakefulness?

Unlike the treatment for those sleep disorders causing profound sleep disturbance and excessive daytime sleepiness, such as obstructive sleep apnoea and periodic leg movements in sleep, requiring direct intervention with sleep itself (Chap. 9), the most effective, long-term treatment of insomnia lies in dealing with the waking day, its problems and stresses, which in turn lead to further worries and distorted beliefs about sleep, with subsequent nocturnal awakenings and lying there ruminating about what the following day portends. To these ends, insomnia is really a 24-hour problem affecting both waking and sleeping life. That is, insomnia is more of a disorder of wakefulness intruding into sleep, rather than one of sleep, and a key focus for CBT-i.

It could be argued that insomnia is more of a natural adaptation of sleep to what life was like many centuries ago, when sleep was a vulnerable state in a more hazardous world. Moreover, a single, long, uninterrupted nighttime period of seamless sleep, which we have come to accept as 'normal' today, is only a comparatively recent development in our history, when less than two hundred years ago, nighttime sleep was typically broken by at least one period of wakefulness in the small hours, often lasting half an hour or so, maybe to eat, add wood to a fire, check one's security, say prayers etc. Roger Ekirch, in his book, *At Day's Close: A History of Nighttime* [17] devotes a whole chapter to this topic, and what we would call today, as 'broken sleep' at night, was typical throughout Europe, and referred to in the English language as 'first' and 'second' or 'morning' sleep, with each country having comparable terminologies. This first sleep usually lasted 2–3 hours broken at around 2 a.m. with this purposeful wakefulness, followed by 3–4 hours of second sleep.

A more contemporary perspective is that one hears about the 'the burden of insomnia in the workplace' and how it may contribute towards absenteeism, rather than the reverse; that is, how the workplace and home life may well be the cause of the insomnia. But usually this is a two-way process, leading to a vicious circle, often leading to what is called poor 'presenteeism' at work, rather than absenteeism, whereby work output is unsatisfactory to all concerned, and maybe eventually leading to work 'burnout' [18], being an inability to work, often lasting for many months. Given that CBT-i is not always readily available from the UK National Health Service, confidential interventions by company occupational health specialists to provide CBT-i, for example, may well be cost-effective in providing for more fully productive staff and better presenteeism, and in minimising absenteeism.

1.13 Tiredness

I mentioned that many people with insomnia feel tired much of the time, despite the hyperarousal, which they largely attribute to their inadequate sleep. This seems rather a contradiction, especially if 'tired' is seen to be synonymous with 'sleepy', which, as I mentioned (Sect. 1.6), does not seem to be the case when sufferers are assessed by sensitive tests of sleepiness, and treatment with hypnotics does not seem to relieve this tiredness. So what is the explanation? People use the word 'tired' within many more contexts than 'sleepy'. This tiredness is not sleepiness, that is a need for sleep, but rather it is a feeling of exhaustion, fatigue, weariness and being worn out, often due to pressures of one's waking life, coupled with too many ruminating thoughts during day and night, especially when trying to get to sleep, which in turn can lead to that 'sleep state misperception' (Sect. 1.6). A good illustration of this confusion comes from a well-known, but in my opinion ambiguous, sleepiness scale, the Stanford Sleepiness Scale (SSS) [19], designed to assess one's sleepiness as it is felt at that moment, and quite distinct from the ESS described earlier, that assesses sleepiness retrospectively. For the SSS the individual has to register one of the following seven questions, seemingly indicating increasing sleepiness:

1. *Feeling active*, vital, alert, wide awake.
2. *Functioning at high level but not peak*, able to concentrate.
3. Relaxed, awake but not fully alert.
4. *A little foggy, let down.*
5. *Foggy*, beginning to lose track, difficult to stay awake.
6. Sleepy, *prefer to lie down, woozy.*
7. *Almost in reverie*, cannot stay awake, sleep onset imminent.

Given its name and what the SSS appears to measure, the words I have shown in itallics in the scale do not necessarily imply sleepiness, but relate to looser feeling states such as 'tiredness', 'malaise', 'lethargy' or 'fatigue', which have much broader lay and clinical interpretations. For example, 'not at peak', 'foggy' or a 'little foggy' do not necessarily mean that one is sleepy. So a tired person may focus on the underlined words, and inasmuch as they might feel 'foggy' this might indicate to whoever is administering the questionnaire that the person is at level 5 and is indeed somewhat sleepy, when they are not. This is probably why for those with insomnia there is little correlation between the score on this scale and the objective measures of sleepiness such as from a reaction time test and the MSLT I described earlier. That is, from the SSS they might register '6' on the scale, apparently declaring sleepiness, but are unlikely to fall asleep as they are wide awake in terms of those objective tests, owing to their hyperarousal, and might just prefer to lie down because they are 'tired'. I should add, again, that arguably the best subjective and unambiguous measure of sleepiness is the Karolinska Sleepiness Scale [20] (Sect. 8.4).

Another example of this semantic problem, but with normal sleepers, is that grogginess, otherwise known as 'post sleep inertia', can last for some hours after sleeping to excess at a time of day when we are normally awake. Whereas a short nap of around 15 minutes is fine, as it comprises only fairly light sleep, and is refreshing within a few minutes of waking up, if this sleep continues for an hour or so, to develop into a full-blown sleep, then it creates a form of temporary 'jet lag' and thick-headedness, due to sleeping more profoundly and out of synchrony with one's usual body clock, which expects one to be awake. Moreover, as some of one's daily sleep need has been obtained in this lengthy nap, it will be more difficult to sleep at night. Nevertheless, someone with this inertia completing the SSS even an hour or so afterwards, will probably respond with a '6', in feeling 'woozy and preferring to lie down'. That is, they seem to be sleepy, but if they were to undergo a MSLT or reaction time test, they would be deemed to be quite alert, albeit 'tired'. On the other hand, by sleeping every afternoon for an hour or so, as in a regular siesta, it becomes part of one's normal daily sleep pattern and the body clock adjusts to it, without that grogginess. Bedtime will be later and night sleep shorter, usually by well over an hour, as daily sleep distributed in this way summates to less sleep overall, and is probably the more 'natural' way of sleeping, rather than one single, longer sleep at night. More about siestas and naps in Sect. 6.6.

A similar semantic problem is seen with other subjective questionnaires apparently relating to 'fatigue', which is also often seen to be synonymous with 'sleepiness'. However, sleep and fatigue can be quite independent of each other [21] as will be seen in the next section.

Interestingly, although 'alertness' and sleepiness might seem to be on the opposite ends of the same dimension, others [22] disagree and have argued that *"subjective states of impaired alertness and excessive sleepiness are independent constructs in the evaluation of sleep-disordered patients"* (p. 258).

To recap, although insomnia is often associated with 'tiredness', which might be assumed to be sleepiness caused by what sufferers perceive to be inadequate sleep, this 'tiredness' is more of a 'mood state', not overcome simply by improving sleep alone, not likely to be due to the insomnia, but a symptom having deeper underlying causes.

Of course, interactions between waking life and insomnia will also depend on personalities. For example, those people having a higher degree of 'perfectionism' will often put excess effort into trying to obtain what they believe has to be more adequate sleep [23], as well as inter-nalise their stress and worries by keeping these emotions to themselves, which may well further aggravate their hyperarousal and insomnia. In these respects they may fall into the category of what their doctors might call the 'worried well'.

Interestingly, in epidemiological studies of insomnia where many respondents have claimed 'tiredness' or 'insufficient sleep', it is often found that these claims seem to reflect a need for more personal 'time-out' rather than for sleep itself. One such study [24] of 12,000 Finnish people aged 33–60 years, reported that 20 % complained of tiredness and/or insufficient sleep. Moreover, a follow-up nine years later, found that almost half of those originally complaining of this were still of the same opinion, and one wonders how they coped with such an ostensibly large accumulated sleep loss, if it existed. However, these respondents also complained of stressful lives, long work hours and poor life satisfaction, and showed signs of depression. That is, simply providing another hour or so of daily sleep was unlikely to be the real solution here, with extra sleep only being one way of achieving more time to oneself, and a topic I pick up again in Sect. 2.2.

1.14 Fatigue

Definitions of 'fatigue' have been the subject of numerous debates, with many conferences and books devoted to the topic. For simplicity, I adopt the more pragmatic interpretation, as a 'decline in performance or attention at any task, whether it be physical or cognitive, due to its prolongation or repetition'. Sleep is not normally required to alleviate it, and in the case of physical fatigue, it is usually just physical rest that is needed, whereas for the fatigue of boredom, it is a more stimulating activity. From the fatigue caused by a cognitively and/or emotionally demanding task, a break is typically needed. Of course, this fatigue is worsened by sleepiness, as well as by the tiredness just described. As 'fatigue' is such a loose and imprecise term, I avoid using it as much as possible.

1.15 Causing Serious Illnesses?

A recent provocative report [25] entitled, 'Does Insomnia Kill?' monitored the health of 13,500 adults, aged between 45 and 69 years, living in North America. Of these, 23 % had complained of insomnia, and over the subsequent six years some died and the others were assessed again. After accounting for various influences such as family income, depressive symptoms, heart and pulmonary disease, neither insomnia nor the use of hypnotics was associated with an increased risk of death. Interestingly, although the prevalence of insomnia is often thought to increase with age, this study also found this not to be the case, after eliminating these other influences.

Other studies have found only tenuous evidence pointing to insomnia as an actual cause of these diseases, rather than the insomnia being just another symptom of something deeper. For example, although insomnia might portend an increased risk for hypertension and cardiovascular disease, for whatever reasons, short sleepers without complaint of insomnia, do not run such a risk [26]. Moreover, simply treating this insomnia alone, maybe with hypnotics, is not known to prevent the development of these diseases.

More serious forms of depression are often accompanied by secondary insomnia, typified by 'early morning awakening', which is used as a diagnostic for this depression. Indeed, links between sleep and depression are strong, with about three-quarters of depressed patients having symptoms of insomnia [26], which is perhaps not surprising given that early morning awakening is a diagnostic for depression. Nevertheless, the evidence is weak that insomnia itself is a substantial cause of depression, especially as it usually takes many years of insomnia before the depression might set in, and the likelihood is that this outcome will not happen anyway [25]. However, the more that people with insomnia believe this potential for depression, the more this could further add to their worries, and become a self-fulfilling prophesy. Besides, sustained attempts to improve this insomnia, by pharmacological methods alone, without dealing with the problems within the individual's waking life (e.g. via CBT-i), are unlikely to offset any eventual depression if it was to materialise [27].

1.16 Summing Up

This chapter has concentrated on the commonest form of insomnia, 'primary' (psychophysiological) insomnia where the cause is largely due to stress and anxieties, and is usually accompanied by hyperarousal. Although the apparently poor sleep, here, can initially be helped with hypnotics, largely as a short-term crutch, more enduring psychological methods, embodied by CBT-i, ought to be utilised, as these have more effective long-term benefits. The extent of sleep loss is not as great as the sufferer usually believes, especially when there is little evidence of excessive daytime sleepiness, as much of this insomnia paradox can be attributed to 'sleep state misperception'. Impairments to waking life, including job performance that is attributed to the insomnia, are unlikely to be simply due to sleep loss, but more to 'tiredness' and/or the hyperarousal. Insomnia by itself does not seem to be the cause of serious physical or mental illnesses, although it can aggravate them, especially when the insomnia is comorbid with pain, for example, thus adding to one's distress, and where the key to dealing with this form of insomnia is to treat the specific causes appropriately. Of course, long-term adjunctive treatments with hypnotics and CBT-i may well be helpful with co-morbid insomnia as well.

The reason why CBT-i and related psychological therapies are the ideal treatment for insomnia, is that insomnia is seen, here, as really a disorder of wakefulness rather than of sleep. Some sufferers fall into the category of the worried well, with the belief that their insomnia will lead to these other illnesses. Apart from this belief being overstated, and even if it turns out to be so, it would probably take many years of sleeping in this manner before such an outcome appeared. Even then it is likely that the insomnia is not the actual cause but part of a vicious circle comprising worry and a poorer quality of both waking life and work satisfaction, often with little real control of one's job, together with limited outside interests and having little time-out for oneself.

References

1. American Association of Sleep Medicine. 2004 Derivation of Research Diagnostic Criteria for Insomnia: Report of an American Academy of Sleep Medicine Work Group. Sleep: 27: 1567–1596.
2. Morin CM et al 2011 The Insomnia Severity Index: psychometric indicators to detect insomnia cases and evaluate treatment response Sleep. 34:601–608.
3. Altena E, et al. 2008 Prefrontal hypoactivation and recovery in insomnia. Sleep. 31:1271–1276.
4. Rosa RR, Bonnet MH 2000 Reported chronic insomnia is independent of poor sleep as measured by electroencephalography. *Psychosom Med*, 62:483–485.
5. Johns MW. 1991 A new method for measuring daytime sleepiness: The Epworth Sleepiness Scale. Sleep 14: 540–545.
6. Edinger JD et al 2008. Psychomotor performance deficits and their relation to prior nights' sleep among individuals with primary insomnia. *Sleep* 31: 599–607.

7. Van Veen MM et al. 2008. Sleep loss affects vigilance: effects of chronic insomnia and sleep therapy. *J Sleep Res* 17:335–343.

8. Roth T et al 2007 Insomnia: pathophysiology and implications for treatment Sleep Med Rev 11: 71–79.

9. Vgontzas AN et al 2001 Chronic insomnia is associated with nyctohemeral activation of the hypothalamic-pituitary-adrenal axis: clinical implications. *J Clin Endocrinol Metab*, 86: 3787–3794.

10. Bonnet MH, Arand DL. 2010 Hyperarousal and insomnia: state of the science. Sleep Med Rev. 14: 9–15.

11. Bonnet MH et al 2014 Physiological and medical findings in insomnia: implications for diagnosis and care. Sleep Med Rev18:111–122.

12. Tworoger SS, et al. 2003 Effects of a yearlong moderate-intensity exercise and stretching intervention on sleep quality in postmenopausal women. Sleep 26: 830–836.

13. Morin CM et al 1999 Nonpharmacologic treatment of chronic insomnia. *Sleep* 22: 1134–1156.

14. Walsh JK et al 2007. Nightly treatment of primary insomnia with Ezopiclone for six months: effect on sleep, quality of life and work limitations. *Sleep* 30: 959–968.

15. Espie CA. 2002 Insomnia: conceptual issues in the development, persistence and treatment of sleep disorder in adults. *Ann Rev Psychol* 53: 215–243.

16. Mitchell CD 2012 Comparative effectiveness of cognitive behavioral therapy for insomnia: a systematic review. *BMC Fam Pract.* 25;13:40.

17. Ekirch R 2005. *At Day's Close- A History of Nighttime.* Kent UK: *Orion Books.*

18. Söderström M, et al 2012 Insufficient sleep predicts occupational burnout. *J Occup Health Psychol* 17:175–183.

19. Hoddes E et al 1973 Quantification of sleepiness: a new approach. *Psychophysiology*, 10: 431–436.

20. Åkerstedt T, Gillberg M. 1990 Subjective and objective sleepiness in the active individual. *Int J Neurosci*;52:29–37.

21. Bailes S et al 2006 Brief and distinct empirical sleepiness and fatigue scales. J Psychosom Res; 60: 605–613.

22. Moller HJ et al 2006. Sleepiness is not the inverse of alertness: evidence from four sleep disorder patient groups Exp Brain Res. 173:258–266.

23. Kales A, et al 1996 Personality patterns in insomnia. Theoretical implications. *Arch Gen Psychiatr*, 33: 1128–1134.

24. Hublin, C et al. 2001. Insufficient sleep – A population-based study in adults. *Sleep.* 24, 392–340.
25. Phillips B, Mannino DM. 2005. Does insomnia kill? *Sleep* 28:965–971.
26. Vgontzas AN et al 2009 Insomnia with objective short sleep duration is associated with a high risk for hypertension. *Sleep* 32: 491–442.
27. Wilson SJ 2010 British Association for Psychopharmacology consensus statement on evidence-based treatment of insomnia, parasomnias and circadian rhythm disorders *J Psychopharmacol.* 24:1577–1601.

2

Sleep Debt: 'Societal Insomnia'?

Long hours of monotonous, uniform work may be endured by men and women without direct physical harm, but at the same time they may render the man unimpressionable to other influences, with incapacity for mental life, all active thought being crushed down to the dull level of monotonous existence...The willing worker, the mechanic interested in completing a job or in his share of the profit, or better still interested in the work, would do more work and keep longer at it without exhaustion than the man without an intelligent interest. A little wholesome competition is enlivening, and acts as a stimulus to work. A promised reward or fear of general failure in a trade, may stimulate individual energy during hours of toil, if there be intelligence and a proper feeling of corporate interest and responsibility. British Medical Journal 1889 'The Labour Question and Hours of Work' (19 October, p. 884).

2.1 Yesterday and Today

The above quote in the abstract comes from the era of Thomas Edison's new electric light, displacing nighttime and helping to create the belief that sleep was just a waste of otherwise valuable work time. In fact, Edison

© The Editor(s) (if applicable) and The Author(s) 2016
J. Horne, *Sleeplessness*, DOI 10.1007/978-3-319-30572-1_2

was quite scathing about what he saw as society's excess of sleep. After all, these were exciting times, with the new industrial age encompassing most of the western world, and ideas that we need 8 hours' sleep or that society was chronically sleep deprived, as is claimed nowadays, were never heard of. Besides, as will be seen, there is little evidence that, today, we sleep fewer hours (maybe a fewer minutes but not hours) than we did then.

A less obvious message, here, is the importance of a wakefulness that is personally fulfilling and worthwhile, providing a desire for more wakefulness and thus less sleep, in contrast with an oppressive wakefulness when more sleep might be a form of retreat. Sleep and mood are intimately linked in a two-way process [1], as even under normal situations when life has its ups and downs, we seem to sleep less when life is going well.

Yet, 'sleep debt' is a contemporary term highlighting concerns that we sleep too little and accumulate a sleep loss that can be too great to reclaim. Furthermore, apart from apparent sleepiness and related safety issues, sleep debt is seen to be a cause of obesity, diabetes, cardiovascular disease and mood changes. Thus, this 'hidden insomnia' seems to be rife in today's society. Added to this apparently lamentable situation are seemingly supportive findings that diabetic-like states can be produced in healthy young adults who have had their sleep restricted to around 4 hours for several nights. More evidence favouring sleep debt comes not only from claims that earlier generations averaged 9 hours' sleep a night, but in beliefs that we rely too heavily on alarm clocks, live in an overworked society, and sleep for longer at weekends simply to repay the previous week's sleep debt. All of which is particularly worrying for those with insomnia, who struggle for even 6 hours of sleep, and whose anxieties are aggravated by the thought of having to strive for even more sleep so as to offset such ill-effects. Needless to say, sleep debt makes a good narrative, attracts much media attention and stokes the demand for sleep aids.

On the other hand, whether we ever slept for longer, or that even 6 hours' daily sleep is really a health risk, are both doubtful, as our sleep duration has actually changed little, certainly not over the last 50 years or so in the UK [2–6]. Where there have been reports of historical reductions in daily sleep, for example, from Scandinavia, these are very small, with 5.5 fewer minutes' daily sleep per 10 years since 1972 [7] but with no change in the proportions of the more extreme sleep durations. In the USA, and in the period between 1975 and 2006, the proportion of adults sleeping fewer than 6 hours a day has increased only by 1.7 % [8]; which is a trend mostly apparent in full-time workers, where working hours have increased little over the years. In contrast, a recent report from the USA [9] found that the incidence of short sleep has decreased by 2 % over the last 30 years. Another report [10] based on the US National Health Interview Surveys conducted in 1985, 1990 and then yearly between 2004 and 2012, covering a total of 324,000 adults (but differing between surveys) found the average decline in sleep duration across these 27 years only to be 13 minutes. So it seems that there has been little recent change in sleep duration, at least in the western world.

Over the years, there have been many short-term laboratory based studies, whereby sleep has been manipulated in some way, for example in assessing the effects of acute sleep restriction, that have often monitored the sleep EEGs of their participants for a few baseline nights beforehand, usually away from home and under the rigours of the laboratory. Although sleep, here, might differ somewhat from at home, this EEG assessment of sleep duration is quite objective. Dr Shawn Youngstedt and colleagues, from various universities in the USA, recently [11] gathered all this fortuitous baseline data from over 250 such studies published between 1960 and 2013, covering a total of 6052 healthy participants aged 18–88 years, who were then divided into 10-year age groups. The investigators found that for none of these age groups had there been any significant change in sleep duration over this more than 50-year period in time. Youngstedt et al. concluded that their findings "challenged the notion of a modern-day epidemic of insufficient sleep" (p. 65).

The basis of claims that we slept for longer, a hundred or so years ago, and in having around 9 hours a night, largely stems from a commonly cited, but misquoted, study centring on the sleep of children and teenagers (aged 6–19 years), not adults [12], which is a topic covered in Chap. 5. More recent claims, for example [13], that in the 1930s, men (not women) used to sleep for longer, are based not on sleep duration itself, but on historic records of people's responses as to whether they felt: 'rested', 'had trouble functioning', 'had stamina', 'were energetic'. That is, these vague terms only allude to excessive sleepiness and sleep loss.

Like other biological characteristics, habitual daily sleep duration in any healthy adult population shows a natural ('normal') distribution, averaging about 7 hours, as can be seen in Fig. 2.1, coming from a fairly recent UK survey [5], of 2000 adult men and women. About two-thirds (plus and minus one 'standard deviation') of this population fell within 1.5 hours either side of this average; that is, two-thirds of these people habitually slept between 5.5 hours and 8.5 hours a night. A larger UK survey [6] of 8500 older adults living in Norfolk, who were aged between 49 and 90 years, found the overall average sleep duration to be 6 hours 50 minutes.

The recent survey from the USA [14] of over 110,000 adults (Fig. 2.2) found a similar range of sleep durations to those of Fig. 2.1, although, as can be seen, the categorisation of durations is less precise.

Of course, apart from naturally occurring short sleepers there are those others who are genuinely chronically sleep deprived, whose sleep falls too short for any adaptation, and who indeed have 'sleep debt'. However, my point is that the prevalence of 'sleep debt' is not so great or alarming as is often claimed, and that the majority of shorter sleepers, especially those habitually sleeping around 6 hours, are usually quite healthy and alert, with little or no sleep debt. Despite claims that short sleep is linked to

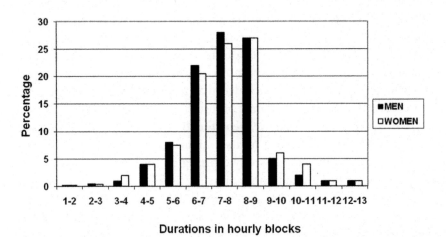

Fig. 2.1 Sleep durations in 2000 UK adults—adapted from Groeger et al. (2004)

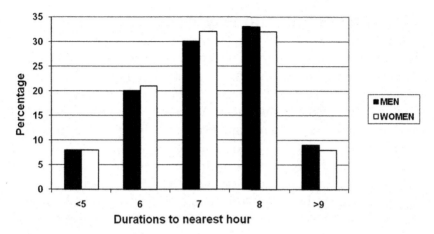

Fig. 2.2 Sleep durations in 110,000 US adults—adapted from Krueger & Friedman (2009)

obesity, it will be seen that this weight gain only really becomes somewhat apparent for those habitually sleeping fewer than 5 hours, whereas it can be seen from both Figs. 2.1 and 2.2, that only around 6 % of adults sleep to this extent.

If, for argument's sake, we did sleep 9 hours at night a hundred or so years ago, then maybe we ought to return to those good old days? Or perhaps not, as life wasn't all so good, then, when, regardless of this sleep people were less healthy, lived fewer years, were shorter in height and poorer. Yet, despite today's 7 hours' sleep we are healthier, live longer, are taller and financially better off. Besides, compare today's sleeping conditions with those of a typical worker a century or so ago, who probably toiled 14 hours daily, six days a week, was likely to live in an impoverished, cold and damp house, and to share a hard and lumpy bed not only with children but with bedbugs and fleas. Arguably those 9 hours comprised fitful sleep. Contrast this with our shorter working week, warm bedrooms, fluffy duvets, contoured pillows and pocket-spring mattresses, when it is likely that 7 hours of uninterrupted quality sleep is just as good, if not better. So, why not spend those 'extra' waking hours being more productive rather than by sleeping? In sum, why attribute sleep in those days as being 'good' for us and that of today being 'bad', when the opposite is likely to be the case?

2.2   Time in Bed and Daytime Naps

Many of today's studies rely on subjective estimates, by asking participants often only a single question concerning the duration of their sleep, which can be poorly defined and often confused with 'time in bed'. It has yet to be shown whether the extent that people misestimate their sleep in this way contains random errors that could simply average out, as is sometimes claimed. Ideally, such data need confirmation more objectively from a 'sleep diary' whereby respondents keep a record for two weeks or so, of times of: going to bed, estimated sleep onset, morning awakening and getting up. But this information is seldom obtained. Moreover, it is important to distinguish between sleep obtained on weekdays (i.e. workdays) and weekends, which have often just been combined. Better still is to use wrist-worn 'actimeters' (see Sect. 2.3), but this method is more costly, and considerably limits the number of participants that can be recruited.

Few discerning comparisons between time in bed and actual sleep duration have been undertaken. One of the best illustrations of the need to distinguish between these two aspects comes from the UK Norfolk survey [6] just mentioned, which reported that the extra time in bed averaged another 1 hour 15 minutes, depending on various factors, especially socio-economic (including work) status, with women spending about 15 minutes longer in bed than men.

Another potential oversight in many of these studies is to overlook daytime naps, or at least 'siestas', as the focus is usually only on nighttime sleep. Their 'cost-effectiveness' in terms of reducing nighttime sleep is described in Sect. 6.2.

2.3   Non-industrial Societies and Seasonal Flexibility of Sleep

Although the industrial age and artificial lighting have been blamed for our declining sleep and today's sleep debt, a remarkable study [15] of three groups of present day native, non-industrial peoples, living without electric light and at various latitudes south of the equator, has come to quite a different conclusion. Two communities live in Africa (latitudes 2° and 20° south) and the other in Bolivia, South America (latitude 15° south). Their lifestyles seem to be influenced by the seasonal differences in daylight (1–2 hours), environmental temperature and food availability. Although only a total of 82 individuals were recruited, their sleep was assessed objectively by each participant wearing a wrist actimeter, continuously for up to 28 days. These devices contain accelerometers that measure arm movement, or rather lack of it, and are good at indicating actual periods of sleep, as it is difficult to keep one's arms still for more than a minute or so when awake. Movements cease with sleep onset, only occurring infrequently during sleep, when shifting the lying position or if waking up during sleep. Movements return quite obviously on eventual morning awakening.

Sleep patterns for all three groups were similar, with sleep being about an hour shorter in the 'summer' compared with the 'winter', with overall averages of 5.7 and 7.1 hours respectively (similar to the seasonal light changes), with the overall average sleep being 6.4 hours, and almost wholly confined to the night. Although waking activity declined under the midday shade, it was unlikely to involve naps as these only occurred on 7 % and 22 % of days in the winter and summer respectively, when naps would last about 30 minutes, to give an overall daily average of this extra sleep of less than 10 minutes. Sleep onset typically occurred about 3–4 hours after sunset, whatever the time of year, but with morning waking closer to sunrise. The authors concluded that as these 'naturalistic' findings in relation to average sleep durations are similar to those of today's western societies, then this argues against present day 'sleep debt' and that we used to sleep for longer.

Another finding [15] from two of these groups, involving much larger samples, was that despite their different cultures and languages, neither group had a word or its equivalent for what we know as 'sleep onset insomnia'. Even when the concept was explained to them in more detail, fewer than 2 % appeared to suffer from it. In the next chapters, it will be seen that short sleep is claimed to be linked to obesity, which was quite absent in these groups and, as the authors also noted, many of these peoples live well into old age.

Another recent and fascinating study [16], comparing two similar hunter-gatherer communities living in northern Argentina (latitude 25° south), but with one group living entirely under natural light and the other with electric lighting, reported similar outcomes in terms of average sleep durations. Again using wrist actimeters worn in the summer and winter, there were seasonal changes to sleep duration. Those without electric light slept about 1.5 hours longer in the winter than summer (about 8.5 versus 7 hours' sleep), and for those with electric light this difference was 1.25 hours (about 7.5 versus 6.25 hours' sleep). Overall, sleep was shorter in the electric light community by about 45 minutes. Of course, for all these native communities, from both studies [15, 16] there would have been seasonal factors apart from light, artificial or natural, for example, the different availabilities and locations of foods. Moreover, electric lighting, or rather electricity, portends other, non-lighting, changes to lifestyles.

Nevertheless, even with electricity and all its advantages, there are still findings of seasonal variations in sleep duration in certain western societies, albeit under extremes, for example, as found above the Arctic Circle. A study [17] based on subjective accounts of sleep obtained from adults living in Tromsö, Norway (latitude 70° north), with its considerable seasonal differences in daylight, found that people slept about one hour longer during the winter than in the summer, with an overall average of about 7 hours.

All these findings with indigenous communities not only point to an average sleep of close to 7 hours, but that our sleep duration is naturally somewhat flexible, given the time to adapt, and as reflected by these seasonal changes to its duration.

2.4   Needing Versus Desiring More Sleep

There have been many surveys, often of a more popular nature, aimed at assessing the extent of 'sleep debt'. Unfortunately, all too many simply rely on what might seem to be the straightforward question, 'would you like to have more daily sleep?' Many people will respond with a 'yes', with the implication that indeed they have sleep debt. But this is a leading question and invites a positive response, as will 'would you like more pay', 'longer vacations' and so on? But how many of us are prepared to forgo time and effort in achieving these ends, including in taking more sleep?

We [18] investigated this apparent desire for more sleep by using more indirect questioning methods. Almost 11,000 adults completed our simple but more discerning questionnaire that avoided leading questions but asked: the times usually going to sleep at night and wake up next morning (from which we calculated usual sleep length); how much sleep they wanted each night (i.e. desired sleep length), their general level of daytime sleepiness, from using the Epworth Sleepiness Scale [19] (ESS—see Sect. 9.2), and whether they had a stressful lifestyle. Of particular importance was that we wished to gauge their resolve in obtaining such extra sleep, and so we then asked, 'if you had an extra hour in the day, how would you prefer to spend it?' Several alternatives were given from which to choose, these being: playing sport or exercising, socialising, reading or relaxing, watching TV or a film, listening to radio, working, sleeping or 'other'.

Women had a greater desire for more sleep than did men, in wanting an average of 8.0 hours versus 7.37 hours' sleep as was the case for men. Nevertheless, when we assessed the differences between actual and these desired sleep durations, to give an apparent sleep deficit, this averaged 25 minutes for men and 29 minutes for women, which were not large amounts. However, the other outcomes were more surprising, especially as we might have expected that the larger this apparent sleep deficit, the greater would be the daytime sleepiness. But this was not so, as there was no such relationship for any age group, for neither men nor women. Moreover, irrespective of the size of this apparent deficit, and with around 50 % of our participants seeming to desire more sleep, at least to some extent, only 20 % of the latter opted to take the extra sleep option rather than those alternative waking activities, even those who were more likely to report moderate or greater levels of daytime sleepiness. It seemed that wanting more sleep was not necessarily synonymous with actually taking more sleep, but in seeming to want more time to oneself, which was largely associated with a more 'stressful lifestyle'. Again, it can be seen that extra sleep may not be the only anodyne for an apparent sleep deficit.

Inasmuch as we also found that young adults sleep longer than older adults, with women sleeping longer than men, these findings reflected similar outcomes from other more general population studies of sleep, e.g. [3, 4], indicating that our sample population was not unusual. In general, women, here, were rather more likely to choose that extra hour for sleeping (23% versus 19% for men), but according to the ESS, women were no sleepier than men, with similar average ESS scores, which were also typical of the population at large, as reported by other investigators. Overall, we found that these apparent sleep deficits did not change with age, although rather more of the younger groups opted for the extra hour in sleeping (men: 18 % for younger versus 15 % for older; women: 24 % versus 19 % for older).

Finally, in a subsequent, much smaller study of ours [20], 43 healthy young adults had their sleep monitored for a week, at home, by using wrist actimeters. We had previously asked them how much sleep they needed, with the difference between this and the recorded sleep giving an indication of the extent of any apparent sleep debt. Despite the range in this debt, it bore no relation with our measures of their daytime sleepiness, as determined by the MSLT and reaction time testing, as well as by the ESS. We concluded that factors other than sleepiness seem to influence these apparent sleep deficits.

2.5   Gender

The sleep durations in Figs 2.1 and 2.2 are not detailed enough to reflect findings that women tend to sleep for around 15 minutes longer than men, which is more apparent in those younger than 45 years of age, and has been reported in a variety of studies, including ours [5], as well as from UK National Statistics. This is not because of myths relating to 'more delicate constitutions', but may well be due to women having more deep or slow wave sleep (SWS—as identified by 'delta' EEG activity—see Sect. 6.1), and a sign of their having greater brain (i.e. cortical) recovery during sleep. This in turn indicates that women tend to work their cerebral cortices harder than the age-related man. Women seem to multitask to a greater extent than men, which requires dealing with information from different sources and senses, then selecting which piece of information to attend to and what to ignore, including having quickly to decide on actions and priorities; all of these are cortically demanding and create much 'brainwork' than, say, reading, completing a crossword, or undertaking tasks sequentially during the day, or having all one's attention focused on a computer screen. Coincidentally or otherwise, maybe owing to a greater degree of 'use it or lose it', and that women happen to retain more SWS with age, the female cortex also ages more slowly than that of men, by about 5 years. So, by the healthy age of 75, the cognitive ability of the female brain is comparable with that of a 70 year old man. More about this 'brainwork' in Chaps. 10 and 11.

Although twice as many women as men consult their doctors about insomnia or other sleep problems, this may be a result of men being more reluctant to go and seek help. Or maybe the women's sleep is more likely to be disturbed by their male partner rather than vice versa? This is not only because snoring is more frequent in men but, for example, in a double bed, the movements of the heavier partner will rock and disturb the other, lighter one, to a greater extent

2.6   For Better or For Worse?

There is a widespread belief that in western countries life today is busier, with greater constraints on sleep time. Although a wide variety of new findings, described in a comprehensive review [21] of our daily use of time over the last 60 years, does not specifically include sleep time, it seems that work hours have not changed. In contrast, leisure time has increased somewhat, but there is little support that we are 'working harder', cf. [21]. We tend to overestimate the time we spend working (including in the USA), and that those who work longer hours tend to overestimate the most, cf. [21]. However, these conclusions exclude two demographic groups: single working parents and "well educated professionals, especially those with small children" cf. [21]. Interestingly, the latter "includes many of the academics who study and discuss the phenomenon" cf. [21]. Of course, nowadays, it is a 'badge of honour' to state that one is busy.

If we did sleep for longer a century or so ago, then why not reverse this perspective and argue that our ostensibly shorter sleep today is fine for us, even more 'natural'? Since in those days if people did sleep for longer they were probably none the better for it, as so many aspects of life were different, being under conditions that few of us today would wish to revert to. Finally, merely to judge sleep by quantity, to the exclusion of its quality presents only a limited perspective on the need for sleep. Besides, from the few 'naturalistic' studies of seasonal changes to sleep, it is apparent that our sleep duration is somewhat flexible. That is, there is a range of quite tolerable 'biological adaptability' within our sleep, just like there is in most, if not all, of our other biological functions.

References

1. Vanderkerckhove M & Cluydts R 2010 The emotional brain and sleep: an intimate relationship. *Sleep Med Rev.*14:219–26.
2. McGhie A, Russell SM. 1962. The subjective assessment of normal sleep patterns. *J Mental Sci* 108: 642–654.
3. Tune GS. 1969. The influence of age and temperament on the adult human sleep-wakefulness pattern. Br J Psychol 60, 431–441.
4. Reyner LA, Horne JA. 1995. Gender and age differences in sleep, determined by home recorded sleep logs and actimetry. *Sleep* 18: 127–134.
5. Groeger JA 2004 Sleep quantity, sleep difficulties and their perceived consequences in a representative sample of some 2000 British adults. *J Sleep Res* 13: 359–371.
6. Leng Y et al 2014. Self reported sleep patterns in a British population cohort. Sleep Medicine 15: 295–302.
7. Kronholm E et al 2007 Trends in self-reported sleep duration and insomnia-related symptoms in Finland from 1972 to 2005: a comparative review and re-analysis of Finnish population samples. J Sleep Res 16: 54–62.
8. Knutson KL. 2010 Trends in the prevalence of short sleepers in the USA: 1975-2006. *Sleep* 33, 37–45.
9. Bin YS et al 2013 Sleeping at the limits: the changing prevalence of short and long sleep durations in 10 countries. *Am J Epidemiol*;177: 826–833.
10. Ford ES et al 2015 Trends in self-reported sleep duration among US adults from 1985 to 2012. *Sleep* 38:829–832.

11. Youngstedt SD et al. 2016. Has adult sleep duration declined over the last 50+ years? *Sleep Med Rev.* 28: 65–81.
12. Terman LM, Hocking A. 1913. The sleep of schoolchildren: its distribution according to age and its relation to physical and mental efficiency. *J Educ Psychol* 4, 138–147.
13. Bliwise, D. 1996 Historical change in the report of daytime fatigue. *Sleep* 19, 462–464.
14. Krueger PM, Friedman EM. 2009 Sleep duration in the United States: a cross-sectional population-based study. *Am J Epidemiol* 169, 1052–1063.
15. Yetish G et al 2015. Natural sleep and is seasonal variations in three pre-industrial societies. *Current Biology*, 25:2862–2868.
16. De la Iglesia HO et al 2015. Access to electric light is associated with shorter sleep duration in a traditionally hunter-gatherer community. *J Biol Ryhthms*, 30: 342–345.
17. Kleitman N, Kleitman H. 1953. The sleep-wakefulness pattern in the Arctic. *Scientific Monthly*, 76, 349–356.
18. Anderson C, Horne JA. 2008. Do we really want more sleep? A population-based study evaluating the strength of desire for more sleep. *Sleep Med*, 184–187.
19. Johns MW. 1991 A new method for measuring daytime sleepiness: The Epworth Sleepiness Scale. *Sleep* 14: 540–545.
20. Anderson C et al. 2009. Self reported 'sleep deficit' is unrelated to daytime sleepiness. *Physiol Behav.* 96:513–517.
21. Pearson H. 2015 The time lab – why does modern life seem so busy? Nature 526:492–496.

3

Short Sleep, Mortality and Illness

Not everything that can be counted counts, and not everything that counts can be counted.

(Albert Einstein)

3.1 Overstated

In continuing the theme 'how much sleep do we really need', the following two chapters focus on the growing numbers of epidemiological studies reporting correlations between habitually short sleep and the increasing likelihood of death, cardiovascular disease, obesity and obesity related disorders. I mentioned earlier (Chap. 1), that this can also be of concern to those with insomnia who might be further worried about these apparent consequences of their not having 'enough sleep'. These correlations should be considered just that, as correlations; not only is it likely that habitually short sleep is just another symptom of deeper, common underlying causes of these health problems, but if short sleep was a cause (amongst others), then in the majority of cases it is not sufficiently strong enough to be of great clinical concern (unless there is

© The Editor(s) (if applicable) and The Author(s) 2016
J. Horne, *Sleeplessness*, DOI 10.1007/978-3-319-30572-1_3

excessive daytime sleepiness), as will be seen. More to the point, there is little or no evidence that longer sleep by itself would rectify these health problems. Rather than spending more time asleep in order to alleviate or prevent obesity, cardiovascular disease and other diseases, there are far more rapidly effective and well-proven treatments, such as a better diet, more exercise and, in many cases, adopting a less stressful lifestyle.

Another issue concerns what it meant by 'habitually short sleep', as the definitions vary and are imprecise. Some studies assume this to be anything below a habitual sleep of 7 hours, whilst others see this to be below 6 hours. Conversely, 'long sleep', which is also associated with somewhat similar physical disorders, has been seen as habitually sleeping beyond 9 or 10 hours. But this often includes those people undiagnosed with major sleep disorders such as obstructive sleep apnoea (Sect. 9.3). Again, it must be appreciated that simply rating sleep on its apparent duration, overlooks the quality of this sleep and degree to which it is disturbed, which are critical factors, unable to be assessed by the majority of these 'field studies' undertaken often via telephone surveys, beyond the clinic or laboratory.

3.2 Clinically Significant?

Many the epidemiological studies of sleep duration and health, reporting highly statistically significant correlations, can be rather misleading in terms of the magnitude of the association, otherwise known as 'effect size'. Even very small correlations of great statistical significance derived from hundreds, maybe thousands of participants, can be too small to be of actual 'clinical significance' or of real practical relevance when compared with other factors. It is all too easy to assume that clinical and statistical significances are synonymous terms, when it is more likely they are not. Unfortunately, in the case of short sleepers, such statistical findings can further buttress the apparent hazards of 'sleep debt', as will be seen. This problem of the assumed equivalence of statistical and clinical significance is found in many other areas of medicine, and when such statistical findings are reported, often of immediate interest to the media and then embellished, they can easily lead to unwarranted worries by the public at large.

Although 'confidence intervals' are often provided with these statistical outcomes, giving a range of values to back up the statistical outcome, in effect these are just a rather different way of expressing the same statistical finding and also easily misinterpreted. A more enlightening and intuitive approach as to whether a finding has 'real meaning', known as Bayesian statistics, involves making an informed guess in advance of a study, not so much by statisticians, but by those who are familiar with the area in question, as to what level of effect or difference could be regarded as of practical or actual clinical interest. Bayesian methods usually have much more discerning criteria as to what is actually 'significant' but, unfortunately, this logically sound approach is seldom used, as critics find it 'too imprecise'.

Another aspect of statistical interpretation, used by many epidemiological studies, is 'odds ratio' (OR), used to describe, for example, the likelihood of short sleepers becoming obese, hypertensive, or developing other medical conditions. Depending on how ORs are determined, the prevalence of a disorder of, say, 25 % in a sample population, versus 75 % for those without it, gives odds of 1:3. If this prevalence doubles to 50 %, giving odds of 1:1, the OR becomes 3, achieved by dividing the odds of 1:3 by 1:1, and giving an impression that the incidence has trebled when it has only doubled. Thus ORs can unwittingly inflate the risk, sometimes considerably [1]. An alternative, somewhat better calculation is 'relative risk' (RR) which cannot always be made owing to the design of the study. RRs are usually more logical and interpretable [1], albeit also a ratio. For example, if the incidence of obesity in a population is 10 % and then doubles to 20 % then the RR is 2 (i.e. divide one by the other), and if to 30 % the RR is 3 and so on. But even this can be misleading, as if this incidence of obesity was instead, only 1 %, and increased to 2 % or 3 % then the RRs would still be 2 and 3 respectively. Which might seem alarming at face value, except that 98 % or 97 % of this latter population are not obese. The simple solution is to give the actual percentages ('absolute risk') and then the reader can decide for themselves. Unfortunately, too many findings fail to provide this information.

3.3   Rounding Up and Down

Most of these studies categorise sleep durations given by respondents into bands, such as sleeping fewer than 5 hours, between 5 and 6 hours, 6 to 7 hours, and so on, which also introduces 'noise' when rounding up or down to the nearest hour, and can be half an hour or more adrift. For example by using such a categorisation, someone sleeping 5.75 hours is sleeping only half an hour less than another person sleeping 6.25 hours, although it might seem that the difference is an hour. Moreover, combining everyone who sleeps fewer than 7 hours as a 'short sleeper' and comparing them with those people sleeping 7–8 hours easily introduces much imprecision, cf. [2]. In contrast, the calculation of obesity, or rather body mass index (BMI), with which sleep is compared, is far more precise, as BMI is derived from body weight in kilograms divided by height, in metres squared, with most people knowing their measurements fairly well. For example, someone weighing 80 kg and with a height of 1.65 m has a BMI of 29.4.

It is often found that there is a significant difference in some 'adverse measure' between those sleeping fewer than 7 hours and those above this amount. Clinically speaking, not only might this be a very small difference, but then the assumption is made that people sleeping fewer than 7 hours are more likely to develop this problem, which is quite unlikely for those sleeping 6–7 hours, albeit somewhat more for those sleeping less than 5 hours. Taking BMI again, which is dealt with in more detail in the next chapter, a greater BMI is more evident in those sleeping fewer than 5 hours, but these sleepers only comprise about 6 % of the population (see Sect. 2.1). Simply combining together everyone sleeping fewer than 7 hours, including those sleeping 6–7 hours, where there is no solid evidence that this will lead to obesity, but which might be so for those sleeping less than 5 hours, then by implication the same applies to the former group. Besides, it will be seen that we still do not know the extent to which this 'short sleep' is a real cause of obesity, even for 5-hour sleepers. Clearly, combining everyone together like this is ill-advised. Also, it will be remembered (Sect. 2.2) that 'time in bed' is often seen to be synonymous with 'time asleep' when the two can differ quite markedly [3].

3.4 Mortality

By far the largest survey to monitor death rates according to sleep duration was by Dr Dan Kripke and colleagues [4], based on the American Cancer Survey of all-cause mortality among 1.1 million adults, monitored for about 10 years. Death was lowest for 6.5–7.5 hour sleepers, compared with 1-hour sleep bands above and below this amount. Interestingly, and later, Kripke and colleagues [5] argued for the benefits of sleep restriction as a method for decreasing mortality in long sleepers, especially as sleep restriction has antidepressant effects, and can also be effective in treating primary insomnia (cf. Sect. 1.10). Indeed, mental health has an important bearing on long and short habitual sleep durations, but as I have already mentioned with respect to insomnia, there is little by way of solid evidence pointing to 'short sleep' actually causing mental illness [6]. However, most mental illnesses do have an impact on sleep, rather than vice versa.

Although Kripke's large survey has been criticised for various shortcomings [7], their findings have been largely borne out by a variety of further reports. For example, there is the 'Nurses Health Study' [8], involving almost 83,000 female nurses tracked for 14 years, during which time 5409 had died. At the beginning of the study the participants had completed questionnaires covering many aspects of their health, including one question on sleep duration. This was then categorised as: 5 hours or less, 6 hours, 7 hours, 8 hours, 9 hours, 10 hours or 11 hours or more, and using 7 hours' sleep as the norm. The RR for 6 hours' sleep was quite low, at 1.07, (i.e. a 7 % relatively greater risk of dying than for 7 hours' sleep), with RRs for fewer than 5 hours, 8 hours and over 9 hours sleep being 1.15, 1.12 and 1.42 respectively.

Another US study [9] lasting over 10 years, based on almost 10,000 middle-aged and elderly adults, categorised their sleep durations into hourly blocks, from fewer than 5 hours to over 9 hours. Whereas no mortality differences were found between 6-, 7- and 8-hour habitual sleepers for the middle-aged (32–59 years) group, this was the case for the elderly (60–86 years) group. The study was notable in being one of the few that also assessed daytime sleepiness, where no such differences were found between the 6-, 7- and 8-hour sleepers for either age group, but it was greater for the short (fewer than 5 hours) and long (more than 9 hours) sleep groups. Of interest, and for the elderly group only, was that the incidence of depression was particularly high (36 %) in these short sleepers, which was almost three times greater than for the 7-hour group. However, it was not known to what extent short sleep contributed towards this depression or vice versa, or whether both were symptoms of a common deeper cause.

From Australia, an impressively large study [10] of 228,000 adults, averaging 45 years of age, required participants to complete a questionnaire assessing sleep duration and pre-existing health problems, as well as social, economic and demographic factors. They were tracked for five years, from 2006. Compared with 7-hour sleepers the risk of mortality was greater for those sleeping at night for fewer than 6 hours (RR: 1.13), although this was still quite small (i.e. 13 %) an increase. For those sleeping for longer than 10 hours the risk was somewhat greater (RR: 1.26). However, when all those with pre-existing health problems were removed, leaving some 175,000 participants, neither these long nor short sleepers had any greater likelihood of death.

Similar findings are seen in China [11], for adults aged over 35 years, who were monitored for about 16 years. Significantly higher RRs for death mostly from cardiovascular disease, were reported for those sleeping fewer than 5 hours or more than 9 hours. Of note was that complaints of persistent insomnia seemed to be a major contributing factor, appearing to have a greater effect than sleep duration alone. Such a view endorses that by another US group [12], mentioned earlier (Sect. 1.15), who describe how those people with both a self-perceived insomnia and a sleep duration of fewer than 5 hours had a higher risk for hypertension, whereas those sleeping more than 6 hours with or without reported insomnia were not at such a risk. That is, perception of one's sleep as being inadequate, as well as stress, rather than sleep duration alone, were seen to be the underlying factors.

In Japan, another large study [13] of 99,000 adults, tracked for 14 years, recorded over 14,000 deaths from all causes. Compared with 7-hour sleepers, men sleeping as designated by 6-, 5- and 4-hour categories, had RRs of mortality comprising 1.2, 1.6 and 2.3 respectively, being somewhat higher for men and lower for women. However, 4 hours' sleep must be seen as quite abnormal, indicative of severe sleep loss, and suggestive of 'over-working', here.

Several comprehensive reviews integrating these and many other somewhat smaller studies of sleep duration and mortality have been published recently, covering findings from various countries. Although the information on sleep from these studies is almost wholly based on a single question put to participants relating to their sleep duration, the overall conclusions are that the risk of mortality is greater in short and long sleepers, but with the definitions of short and long sleep having various cut-offs from study to study. Nevertheless, and overall, these particular RRs remain low albeit highly statistically significant. For example, in one such review [2] mortality RRs for short sleep were 1.13 for men and 1.07 for women sleeping fewer than 7 hours. Remember, that fewer than 7 hours' sleep is a 'catch all' including those sleeping below 5 hours. Whilst another such review [14] came to a similar conclusion, again by including everyone sleeping fewer than 7 hours, and with similar mortality RRs from assessing the outcomes of 16 studies, the authors conceded that this finding was more likely to be based on those sleeping fewer than 5 hours. A particularly insightful review [15] not only pointed to various possible underlying causes of death in short sleepers, such as cardiovascular disease, obesity, 'stress', poor socio-economic status and living in deprived areas, but it also clarified how short sleep could be linked to, but not necessary cause increased mortality. Two final notable points: at least in older adults, more extreme sleep durations are often associated with self-perceived poorer health, as determined by various physical and mental health questionnaires, cf. [15, 16], and secondly, the possible underlying illnesses associated with short sleep are not necessarily the same as those for long sleepers.

To conclude this topic on mortality and sleep, healthy adults whose habitual daily sleep is 6 hours or thereabouts, should not be concerned that this amount of sleep, alone, is much more likely to cause illness or death than that for 7–8 hour sleepers. Unless of course, there is also excessive daytime sleepiness, where there is the increased risk of a serious accident, These overall findings should be of comfort to most people with insomnia, whose sleep is usually not particularly short, usually totalling around 6 hours in duration when determined (not by themselves) by more objective methods (see Sect. 1.6). Moreover, the study [17] I mentioned earlier (1.15—Does Insomnia Kill?), based on 13,000 participants aged 45–69 years tracked for 6 years, of whom 23 % had insomnia, reported no increase in mortality amongst these sufferers, and neither was their use of hypnotics any riskier.

Other findings showing a greater mortality risk for those sleeping fewer than 5 hours may well be linked to waking pressures and lifestyle factors that also cause short sleep, especially as there is little evidence that their obtaining extra sleep, alone, without supportive therapies such as CBT-i, will rectify these latter problems. Nevertheless, having mentioned all this, there is a link between insomnia and hypertension but, again, this is probably not due to the insomnia itself, as will now be seen.

3.5   Cardiovascular Disease (CVD)

A US National Health Interview Survey of over 110,000 adults [18] asked the single question, "on average how many hours of sleep do you get in a 24h period?" People responded to the nearest hour using the categories: '5 or fewer hours, 6, 7, 8 hours, etc'. Thus '6 hours' extended from about 5.5 to 6.5 hours, with '7 hours' as the norm, although it was actually between 6.5 and 7.5 hours. On this basis, and with comparisons based on the 7 hours, the RR of cardiovascular disease (CVD) and respiratory diseases as well as type 2 diabetes was a statistically significant 1.1 for 6 hours' sleep. However, this 10 % difference between these latter two sleep groups was small in comparison with the greater influence of other factors that had also been collected, such as being African-American, having young children, working long hours and smoking, where all these latter RRs were much greater than 1.1 for this 6-hour sleep group.

In the 'Sleep Heart Health Study' [19] involving almost 6000 US adults, 6–7 hour sleepers had a significantly higher risk of hypertension, compared with 7–8 hour sleepers. However, the difference in mean systolic blood pressure between these two groups was actually very small, only 2.1 mmHg (130.5 versus 128.4 mmHg) and for diastolic pressure it was only 0.7 mmHg (75.0 versus 74.3 mmHg). Neither difference could be considered as 'clinically worrying'. In fact, these averages are under the usual hypertensive thresholds, even for those sleeping less than 6 hours. More to the point is that increasing sleep by an hour or so would be unlikely to lower hypertension where it might exist in short sleepers, whereas spending a portion of this extra hour in walking, instead, is likely to be more effective and therapeutic.

Rather than compare the prevalence of hypertension in short and normal sleepers, a discerning Swiss study [20] of 2162 patients, averaging 58 years of age, compared the sleep durations (as determined by sleep EEGs) of those with and without hypertension. Only a very small difference in sleep of less than five minutes was found between these two groups.

The largest studies on CVD and sleep duration have recently come from Australia [21] involving almost a quarter of a million adults living in New South Wales, whose health records were assessed, together with their responses to 'how many hours in each 24 hour day do you usually spend sleeping?' The number of hours was categorised into hourly blocks upwards from 'under 6 hours', to 'more than 10 hours'. 'Under 6 hours' was significantly associated with CVD (RR: 1.38) compared with 7 hours' sleep. However, a subsequent tracking of other 6-hour sleepers, who seemed to be free of CVD at this time but after some years were subsequently admitted to hospitals with CVD, showed no greater incidence of the disease than for the 7-hour group. I will return to this important study shortly (Sect. 4.4), as it also reported on type 2 diabetes.

A UK study [22] only found a habitual nightly sleep duration of fewer than 5 hours to be associated with a higher risk of CVD, but only for women. This association fell when psychiatric status was included, and no such associations were detected in men. A later analysis by this same group [23], refining the outcome for women, found CVD to be more evident pre-menopausally, even when socio-economic status and psychiatric comorbidities were controlled for.

In order to make better sense of contrasting findings from similar studies, there is a complex statistical technique called 'meta-analysis', that combines all these findings into one large analysis, designed to extract common features and patterns by loading the outcomes from each study according to strict criteria. Nevertheless, meta-analyses can still be liable to biases, depending on the various criteria selected by those carrying out these analyses, and thus can produce somewhat misleading outcomes. Such meta-analyses have been undertaken on reports linking hypertension with sleep duration where, for example [24], short sleep was defined as fewer than 6 hours, and long sleep as over 9 hours. Both durations were compared with 7–8 hours' sleep in terms of the likelihood of hypertension, and resulted in a significant RR of 1.23 for short sleep but not for long sleep. However, this analysis did not discriminate for sleeping between 5 and 6 hours, where it might well be assumed that this risk would have been greater for those sleeping less than 5 hours.

Thus it would seem that at least for those sleeping between 6 and 8 hours there is little by way of any associations with CVD, and certainly not to the extent that one could claim that 6–7 hours' sleep was a real cause, here. However, there are some interesting findings associated with the taking of afternoon siestas (in siesta cultures). Unfortunately, none of these particular studies provided information on nighttime sleep duration. A large and discerning investigation [25] was carried out of over 23,000 healthy Greek adults without history of CVD, stroke or cancer, who were followed-up for six years. Those having a siesta of longer than 30 minutes, taken more than three times a week, were 30 % less likely to die from CVD, especially those who were working. Although siesta takers were less likely to engage in physical exercise, they were more likely to find the siesta 'stress releasing'. Other studies have reported similar effects of siestas, particularly in the elderly [26].

3.6   Breast Cancer

There have been claims that short sleep is associated with breast cancer, but findings are equivocal, as on the one hand, a study [27] of 23,995 women followed for 9 years, found a greater prevalence of breast cancer only in those habitually sleeping fewer than 6 hours compared with separate groupings for 7, 8 and above 9 hours' sleep. On the other hand, a large investigation [28] found about a 6 % increased risk for breast cancer per hour of habitual sleep beyond 8 hours, whereas sleeping fewer than 7 revealed no association.

3.7 Immunity

The immune system comprises many highly intricate, interacting mechanisms. Although 'lack of sleep' can increase vulnerability to infections, with too many late nights leading to colds and influenza and so on, the underlying reason is not necessarily sleep loss itself, but stress, maybe from overwork, for example, with both sleep loss and increased susceptibility to infection being the result of stress. A major factor, here, is an increase in our 'stress coping' hormone, cortisol (see Sect. 1.8) which, rather paradoxically, can also suppress aspects of the immune system.

Laboratory studies of total sleep deprivation, whereby healthy participants are well looked after, are happy and entertained in their free time, are not required to lie down for long periods and then struggle to remain awake, who can withdraw from the study whenever they want, show that the participants suffer little by way of such stress effects [29]. Interestingly, military exercises including sleep loss have found that cortisol levels rise only when there is additional 'battle stress' and/or belief that one will not be able to cope psychologically with the situation [29]. That is, under sleep loss settings, where the individual feels in control, and that this is part of a reasonably acceptable, even enjoyable albeit challenging situation, there is little by way of such a stress response.

Although alterations to the immune system often appear during sleep loss, unrelated to any changes to cortisol output, these are not necessarily sufficiently large enough to impair immunity, even though these changes might be highly statistically significant, implying that this is a failing of immunity. But rather, this may only indicate a harmless, natural boosting or rebalancing of immune responses, merely in preparation for any increased likelihood of exposure to infection from being awake for longer, rather than remaining in one's relatively protected environment of the bed and bedroom. Indeed, an excellent review of sleep and immunity [30] has also pointed out that sleep loss leads only to equivocal changes in human immune function, which are not necessarily detrimental but may simply indicate heightened immunological activity.

Two recent studies looking at sleep duration and immunity [31, 32] again illustrate difficulties here and problems with generalisations. Both exposed healthy volunteers to the cold virus (rhinovirus) and monitored them for 5 days, under quarantine, to see if a cold developed. One [31] reported that those who habitually slept less than 7 hours (by self-report) were 3 times more likely to develop a cold than those sleeping for longer than 8 hours. However, the extent to which, for example, 6–7 hour sleepers were more vulnerable was not reported as shorter sleepers were included. More important was the finding that those with more disturbed and poorer sleep were 5.5 times more likely to develop a cold, regardless of sleep duration. The reasons for these disturbances are unknown.

The second study [32] monitored sleep more objectively during the infection phase, using wrist actimeters (see Sect. 2.3). Participants were isolated for the 5 days in hotel rooms. Interestingly, the majority of participants did not contract actual colds. Whilst 45 % of those sleeping less than 5 hours did so, compared with 17 % for those sleeping longer than 7 hours, for those sleeping between 6–7 it was 23 %, which was not significantly different from the previous group. For those sleeping 5–6 hours this incidence was 30 %. Sleep disturbance was claimed not to be a contributory factor.

Finally, studies of totally sleep-deprived laboratory rodents found a collapse of the animals' immune system, leading to septicaemia and eventual death after about 2 weeks. However, these outcomes must be seen within the context of the extreme, highly unnatural and very restricted conditions for the animals, where I have argued elsewhere that the 'stress controls' are not adequate [29]. Perhaps more remarkable is the resilience of these animals who survive for so long without sleep.

3.8   Wear and Tear

There is little evidence to show that apart from our brain, sleep in adults provides little by way of greater recovery benefit for other organs beyond what happens when just lying relaxed but awake rather than asleep during the night. The monitoring of the functions of these other organs during the night shows no obvious unique benefits of sleep that cannot be achieved during resting wakefulness, apart from a greater slowing down of activities. Breathing and heart rate become more irregular at times during sleep, which is nothing unusual and, for example, kidney, liver and gut show nothing remarkably different. That is, none of these organs 'sleep', other than relaxing somewhat, and do not appear to show essential changes unique to sleep. Claims that our sleep conserves energy are weak [29], as our energy requirement, reflected by total body oxygen consumption, only falls by about 15 % when asleep at night, compared with lying awake. In rough terms, this extra energy saving during 7 hours' sleep only summates to less than 150 Calories for the average adult, which has the energy equivalent of a slice of bread or a handful of peanuts.

Most body cells have a limited life span (excluding, for example, those of the brain and heart), thus die and are replaced by the multiplication of younger cells which have grown to the appropriate size, given adequate nutrients from recently digested food, absorbed from the gut into the blood and thence supplied to these cells. Certain body cells, especially those of the skin, show peaks of cell division (mitosis) in the small hours of the morning, coinciding with slow wave sleep (SWS) and a surge in the output of growth hormone—implying that sleep might indeed promote general growth and repair. However, there is a circadian rhythm in these peaks, due neither to sleep nor to the growth hormone surge, as these peaks remain if one stays awake, adequately fed and relaxed at this time. Another rise in mitosis can be seen a few hours after lunch when resting, but awake. I should add that physical exercise at these times suppresses these peaks, until the ensuing rest period [29].

Skin cells are amongst the most rapidly dividing of body cells, replacing those that are continually being worn off during everyday activities. This includes the facial skin, and although it is often thought that these early morning peaks in mitosis help reduce facial wrinkles, as in 'beauty sleep', this effect is typically short-lived and has little to do with mitosis. Sleep, especially SWS, causes an increase in skin perspiration, especially from the cheeks and forehead, which contain a rich supply of capillaries (hence the ease by which the face can flush from its underlying capillaries dilating with more blood). Such facial flushing, particularly evident in SWS, provides for a relatively high rate of evaporative heat loss from the face, as this is usually the only part of the body exposed to the outside air and, thus, can help keep the body cool during sleep. This causes facial skin to become spongier in sleep, and in doing so causes those wrinkles to flatten out, an effect that is seen when looking in the mirror soon after awakening in the morning. Unfortunately, they soon reappear as the skin dries out. Many 'overnight anti-wrinkle creams' merely reduce this evaporation, slowing down skin drying, keeping it more hydrated during the subsequent wakefulness. As the skin under the eyes is particularly thin, the underlying tissue is more liable to become spongy, causing 'bags' under the eyes on awakening, that soon reduce back into wrinkles. Unfortunately, all this stretching and contraction of the skin can eventually create a greater profusion of these particular wrinkles. 'Brown rings' under the eyes are usually not from chronic sleep loss itself, but tend to be due to the chronic 'tiredness' I described in Sect. 1.13.

Despite it often being thought that sleep, more than just physical rest, facilitates muscle recovery after heavy physical exercise, there is little or no evidence to this effect, and several studies have shown this, as indeed so have we [33]. One way of demonstrating this lack of any specific effect of sleep is to measure the efficiency of working muscle during sleep loss, by monitoring one's oxygen consumption under a fixed physical workload, as in cycling on a bicycle ergometer, for example. This efficiency does not change, even during 3 days without sleep, given adequate physical (non-sleeping) rest [33]. Neither does cardiovascular efficiency, that is heart rate under various workloads, change during sleep loss,. But there are psychological factors to contend with, as sleepy people are often less motivated to persevere with this exercise (i.e. exercise 'endurance' declines), as they are more likely to view the same exercise load to be heavier than usual, despite there being little or no physiological basis for this.

3.9   William Gale

Let me end this chapter on a lighter 'societal' note by returning to the Victorian age. There have been many reports of sustained physical endurance involving considerable sleep loss during successful attempts to break various records. Amongst the earliest were those in the late 1870s, when extreme walking became popular in the UK, particularly with the remarkable feats of stamina by the 45-year-old William Gale, who received considerable newspaper coverage and acclaim, as the 'diminutive pedestrian from Wales'. He walked 1500 miles in 1000 hours, walking for an average of ¼ of a mile every 10 minutes followed by 3–4 minutes of sleep every hour throughout day and night, aided by his reclining in an armchair with his legs elevated (he had varicose veins) during the day or on a couch at night. The British Medical Journal also reported several successive accounts of his progress, mostly given by his doctor, Dr F J Grant (BMJ 10 November 1877, p. 678), who noted that he was a small man, "*5ft 3½ inch tall and weighing 8 stone 7 pounds*", with a "*peculiar placidity of mental disposition … very modest and unassuming*". He indulged in "*a very injudicious diet with regard to food, although abstaining as usual from alcohol*". Initially his food breaks consisted of "*lobster and pickled pork, walnuts and grapes, followed by hot buttered muffins and six cups of tea*". However, thanks to the intervention of Dr Grant, he was subsequently put onto a "*regulated diet*". Four years later he attempted a 2500 mile walk, also in 1000 hours, and almost succeeded only missing the deadline by 95 miles. This was on a circular track and under close medical supervision (BMJ 8 January 1881, p. 62), when he would walk 1¼ miles every half an hour, with intervals for sleep and so on being less than 10 minutes. Towards the end he was walking at night in a "*half conscious state without perfect co-ordination but when spoken to he instantly became conscious*". Medical examination at the end, by Dr Grant, reported nothing unusual apart from drowsiness. There was no joint pain or swelling, and he had lost only 8 pounds in weight. As far as I can tell, nothing more is known about him.

Many other men and some women (called 'pedestriennes', cf. [34]) attempted endurance walking at this time, but not to his extent. Needless to say, this 'suffrage feminism' as it was called by the media of the time, was frowned on, as such exertions were seen to be contrary to women's frailties and an infringement of their virtue. Nevertheless, the most famous of these women was Ada Anderson, a cockney, from the east end of London, who walked many hundreds of miles with minimal sleep, having spent 3 months training with William Gale. However, after finding little support in the UK, she took her walking skills to the USA where she became a celebrity, feted by the media, and inspired many other women to emulate her physical endurances involving little sleep. Her remarkable achievements are well worth a read [34].

References

1. Schmidt CO, Kohlmann T 2008 When to use the odds ratio or the relative risk? *Int J Public Health* 53, 65.
2. Gallicchio L., Kalesan, B. 2009 Sleep duration and mortality: a systematic review and meta-analysis. *J Sleep Res* 18, 148–158.
3. Leng Y et al 2014. Self reported sleep patterns in a British population cohort. Sleep Medicine 15: 295–302.
4. Kripke DF et al 2002. Morality associated with sleep duration and insomnia. *Arch Gen Psychiat* 9, 131–136.
5. Youngstedt SD, Kripke DF. 2004 Long sleep and mortality: rationale for sleep restriction. Sleep Med Rev 8, 159–174.
6. Buysse DJ et al 2010. Can an improvement in sleep positively impact on health? *Sleep Med Rev* 14: 405–410.
7. Buysse D, Ganguli M 2002 Can sleep be bad for you? Can insomnia be good? *Arch Gen Psychiat* 59, 131–136.
8. Patel SR. 2009 Reduced sleep as an obesity factor. *Obesity Rev* 10 (Suppl 2), 61–68.
9. Gangwisch JE et al 2008 Sleep duration associated with mortality in elderly, but not middle-aged, adults in a large US sample. *Sleep* 31, 1087–1096.
10. Magee CA et al 2013 Investigation of the relationship between sleep duration, all-cause mortality, and preexisting disease *Sleep Med*. 14: 591–6.
11. Chien K et al 2010 Habitual sleep duration and insomnia and the risk of cardiovascular events and all-cause death: report from a community-based cohort. *Sleep* 33, 177–184 430.
12. Vgontzas AN et al 2009 Insomnia with objective short sleep duration is associated with a high risk for hypertension *Sleep* 32, 491–497.
13. Ikehara, S et al 2009 Association of sleep duration with mortality from cardiovascular disease and other causes for Japanese men and women: the JACC Study. *Sleep* 32, 259–301.
14. Faubel R et al 2009 Sleep duration and health-related quality of life among older adults: a population-based cohort in Spain. *Sleep* 32, 1059–1068.
15. Cappuccio FP et al 2010 Sleep duration and all-cause mortality: a systematic review and meta-analysis of prospective studies. Sleep 33, 585–592.
16. Grandner MA et al 2010 Mortality associated with short sleep duration: The evidence, the possible mechanisms, and the future. *Sleep Med Rev* 14, 191–203.
17. Phillips B, Mannino DM. 2005. Does insomnia kill? *Sleep* 28:965–971.

18. Krueger PM, Friedman EM. 2009 Sleep duration in the United States: a cross-sectional population-based study. *Amer J Epidemiol* 169, 1052–1063.
19. Gottlieb DJ et al 2006. Association of usual sleep duration with hypertension: the sleep heart health study, Sleep 29, 1009–1014.
20. Haba-Rubio J et al. 2015. Objective sleep structure and cardiovascular risk factors in the general population: the HypnoLaus study. *Sleep*, 38: 391–400.
21. Holliday EG et al 2013 Short sleep duration is associated with risk of future diabetes but not cardiovascular disease: a prospective study and meta-analysis. *PLoS One* 8(11):e82305.
22. Cappuccio FP et al 2007 Gender-specific associations of short sleep duration with prevalent and incident hypertension: the Whitehall II Study. *Hypertension* 50, 693–700.
23. Stranges S et al 2010 A population-based study of reduced sleep duration and hypertension: the strongest association may be in premenopausal women. *J Hypertension* 28, 896–902.
24. Guo X et al 2013 Epidemiological evidence for the link between sleep duration and high blood pressure: a systematic review and meta-analysis. *Sleep Med.* 14:324–332.
25. Naska A et al 2007 Siesta in healthy adults and coronary mortality in the general population *Arch Internal Med* 167, 296–301.
26. Bursztyn M, Stessman, J 2005 The siesta and mortality: twelve years of prospective observations in 70-year-olds. Sleep 28, 345–347.
27. McElroy JA et al 2006 Duration of sleep and breast cancer risk in a large population-based case-control study. *J Sleep Res* 15, 41–49.
28. Kakizaki M et al 2008 Sleep duration and the risk of breast cancer: the Ohsake Cohort study. *Br J Cancer* 99, 1502–1505.
29. Horne JA. 1988. Why We Sleep. Oxford: University Press
30. Bryant PA et al 2004. Sick and tired: does sleep have a vital role in the immune system? *Nature Rev Immunol*, 457–467.
31. Cohen S et al 2009 Sleep habits and susceptibility to colds *Arch Intern Med* 269: 62–67.
32. Prather AA et al 2015 Behaviorally assessed sleep and susceptibility to the common cold. *Sleep* 38: 1353–1359.
33. Horne JA, Pettitt AN 1984 Sleep deprivation and the physiological response to exercise under steady-state conditions in untrained subjects. *Sleep.* 7:168–179.
34. Shaulis D 1999 Pedestriennes - newsworthy but controversial women in sporting entertainment. *J Sport History* 26: 29–50.

4

Obesity

4.1 Lean Times

Sleep debt has been seen not just as a correlate of obesity but as a cause, and further leading to various health problems, particularly the 'metabolic syndrome', often seen as a 'pre-diabetic state'. This comprises a collection of disorders, including a 'pot belly' ('central obesity'), elevated blood pressure bordering on hypertension, high fasting blood glucose levels, and often high blood levels of triglycerides and cholesterol. Both the latter are 'lipids', with triglycerides being a form of energy store, whereas cholesterol is a building block for cells and many of our (steroid) hormones, including cortisol. If not treated, usually by weight loss, this syndrome can eventually develop into the most common form of diabetes (type 2), mainly resulting in excessively high blood sugar levels (hyperglycaemia) mostly due to insufficient insulin being available to reduce these levels, and known as 'insulin resistance' or 'glucose intolerance'.

Seemingly, this sleep debt related obesity with its metabolic consequences are not necessarily due to excessive sleepiness, indolence and a lesser inclination towards exercise, but to the more subtle effects of insulin resistance [1]. Other hormones regulating feeding behaviour and

© The Editor(s) (if applicable) and The Author(s) 2016
J. Horne, *Sleeplessness*, DOI 10.1007/978-3-319-30572-1_4

metabolism, notably leptin and ghrelin can also be affected by severe sleep loss or, more to the point, by acute sleep restriction in healthy adults, as I will come to shortly. Leptin is a satiety hormone released by fat cells, not only telling the brain to stop us from eating, but it regulates the amount of body fat that is stored. On the other hand, ghrelin is a hunger hormone produced by the empty stomach, encouraging us to eat. Although seeming to work in opposite ways, these hormones have more complex effects on the body's overall use of its energy reserves, collectively known as 'energy balance'.

The reason for my explaining all this is that several laboratory studies, e.g. [2], on healthy, lean young adults having had their night sleep restricted usually to 4 hours for several nights, found changes indicative of the 'metabolic syndrome'. That is, changes to insulin resistance, and to leptin and ghrelin levels which, together, increase hunger and appetite. These effects soon disappear when the participants have up to 10 hours recovery sleep for a couple of days. Not surprisingly, these findings have attracted much attention and are frequently used to buttress claims that sleep debt is a cause of metabolic syndrome and obesity, with longer sleep in short sleepers potentially being a novel behavioural intervention to prevent weight gain or facilitate weight loss, e.g. [3].

However, such levels of extreme and sudden sleep restriction are usually stressful, as participants are confined to bed throughout the night, with their restricted sleep maintained by the 'gentle assistance' of helpers. Of course, participants become extremely sleepy during this regimen, as no one can adequately cope with only 4 hours' sleep per night, sustained over several days, and the stress can lead to a rise in cortisol, which itself impairs glucose tolerance. Interestingly, these latter findings with sleep restriction are particularly evident when compared with the subsequent recovery days, and to a lesser extent when compared with the previous (baseline) days, when participants had slept normally. As cortisol levels are very much governed by one's perception of a stressful event, then any apprehension on behalf of the participants during baseline will cause these levels to rise, worsen during the restriction, maybe followed by feelings of relief on recovery days and accompanied by a fall in cortisol. This cortisol 'dynamic' may well contribute to these findings with glucose tolerance, as a participant's 'state of mind' is so important in these studies, so easily overlooked when other more tangible physiological methods are monitored.

In effect, 4 hours' sleep over several days is intolerably short and psychologically stressful. Outside the laboratory, in the real world, so very few people can sleep as little as this, as was seen in Chap. 2. Thus, it is unclear to what extent these findings can be generalised to those people who habitually sleep, say 6 hours a night (even to 5-hour sleepers) who, despite being identified as having 'sleep debt', may well be leading healthy and happy lives. So we must be cautious in interpreting these experimental studies, where the greatest health risk of sleeping only 4 hours a day is excessive daytime sleepiness and the risk of injury, or worse, especially when driving.

Sleep quality and quantity are a litmus test for a variety of physical and psychological disorders and problems, and any association between short sleep and obesity is more likely due to common underlying causes. Moreover, and as will be seen, any sleep-related real risk of an adult becoming obese or overweight is not apparent until habitual sleep is down to around 5 hours per 24 hours which, as already noted, comprises only a small minority of the population. If, say, 7 hours' sleep a day is advocated as the norm, then the apparent 2-hour shortfall in sleep for the 5-hour sleeper accumulates to over 700 hours of 'lost' sleep annually. In contrast, the weight gain that could specifically be attributed to this 5-hour sleep over a year accumulates to less than 2 kg which can be worked off in very much shorter periods of daily brisk walking, apart from having a calorie restrictive diet. That is, only about 15 minutes of the time within that potential extra 2 hours' sleep would be needed for brisk walking in order to produce the same notional weight loss over a year—totalling around 90 hours of brisk walking versus that 700 hours of extra sleep.

If, instead, one was to argue that hypnotics, and other sleep aids should be considered as 'dietary supplements' for helping obese short sleepers to extend their sleep in an attempt to lose weight, such methods would unlikely to work as, noted earlier (Sect. 1.9), few prescribed hypnotics taken for more than a matter of weeks will extend sleep by more than 30 minutes, despite improving sleep onset.

4.2   Body Mass Index (BMI)

There are ever increasing numbers of studies finding significant associations between short sleep and BMI which, it will be remembered (Sect. 3.3), is calculated as weight in kilograms divided by height in metres squared. Before describing some of these more pertinent findings, let me give some background to this index, used universally as a guide to obesity, despite its limitations. First devised in 1832 by the Belgian polymath, Adolphe Quetelet in his quest to define the 'normal man', it became known as the Quetelet Index, but was renamed as BMI in 1972 by Ancel Keys, a renowned physiologist. One of BMI's shortcomings is that very muscular people can have a high BMI, indicative of obesity, when they are in fact quite lean. This is why waist circumference is a useful additional measure of 'pot bellyness' and clearly an index of obesity, as well as being more indicative of the metabolic syndrome. Whereas the normal range for BMI is between 18.5 and 25, a BMI between 26 and 29 is deemed as 'overweight', 30 and above classified as 'obese', with the latter's sub-division of 30–34 viewed as 'grade 1 obesity'. However, these rather arbitrary boundaries were originally set many years ago, just after the Second World War and, in all senses, during 'leaner times'. Thus, the extent to which these cut-off points are indicative of levels of 'unhealthiness' in today's society, especially within the 'overweight' category, remain a matter for debate. What if, for example, it was decided that the naturally healthy state for humans is to be a bit fatter than, say, 50 years ago, when people tended to be less healthy and had a somewhat shorter life expectancy? If, say, the BMI cut-off for being overweight was shifted upwards by a couple of points, then at a statistical stroke, millions of people deemed to be overweight would now be of normal weight.

However, in 1998, the US National Institutes of Health lowered the BMI 'overweight' threshold from 27.8 to 25 to match international guidelines, but it had little scientific proof with which to support this reduction. Nevertheless, evidence favouring the higher threshold came in 2013, from a controversial paper [4] by Dr Katherine Flegal and colleagues, from the US National Center for Health Statistics, published in the prestigious Journal of the American Medical Association. Covering a large number of studies that together included 2.88 million adults, of whom around 270,000 had died, the investigation undertook a series of discerning analyses to produce 'hazard ratios' (HRs—similar to relative risks—see Sect. 3.2) of the chances of dying if one is overweight or obese. By using the 'traditional BMI boundaries' of 25 and 30, compared with the normal range, the outcome from this study was surprising, as being 'overweight' was not associated with a greater likelihood of death, but marginally safer, with a HR of under 1 (HR: 0.94). For what the investigators called 'grade 1 obesity' (BMI between 30 and 34) this outcome was still no different (HR: 0.95), but rose (HR: 1.29) for BMIs of 35 and above. Needless to say the paper caused a furore. I will avoid this debate but simply note that being overweight, even somewhat obese, is not necessarily a health hazard for everyone as they can be 'fat and fit'. In fact, for elderly people there is what is called 'paradoxical obesity' where moderate obesity can enhance survival with certain disorders such as cardiovascular disease.

Nevertheless, this issue of BMI cut-offs points to differences in medical opinion about the clinical relevance of what can be small differences in BMI. More to the point, the findings relating BMI to habitual durations of sleep are often claimed to be of much greater clinical relevance than might otherwise be the case.

4.3 Population Studies

There are two broad categories of studies, here. A 'case-control' study takes a 'snapshot' of the present status of a large population and, for example, assesses each participant's estimated sleep duration with their BMI, including various other factors apart from age and gender, such as socio-economic status, education, etc. It would then compare the various sleep durations in terms of BMI. The second type of investigation is a 'prospective cohort' study which takes similar measures, but follows individuals for some years to see how BMI might change over time in comparison with their sleep. These two approaches are not exclusive, as by taking snapshots during the course of a cohort study and comparing these sleepers, both aims are achieved.

There are many findings to choose from [cf. 4], but as the conclusions are similar I will select those that illustrate key points. The prospective 'Nurses Health Study' I mentioned earlier (Sect. 3.4), also measured [5] body weights (but not BMIs) over a 16-year period, in 68,183 female nurses, and found for each year measured, that those who reported sleeping fewer than 5 hours consistently weighed more than those sleeping longer than this amount. In the first year of the study, those categorised as sleeping fewer than 5 hours, or 6, 7 and 8 hours were all similar in weight, weighing respectively 69.7 kg, 68.4 kg, 67.1 kg and 67.8 kg, although the shortest sleepers were somewhat the heaviest. Sixteen years later, despite all groups gaining weight and the shortest sleepers remaining heavier, the latter group's overall weight gain was only 2.8 kg more than for the 7-hour sleepers, and 3.2 kg more than for the 8-hour sleepers (the actual weight increases being 7.6 kg, 5.9 kg, 4.8 kg and 4.4 kg respectively). These differences were despite what might well have been a 10,000-hour potential accumulated difference in sleep durations between the 5- and 7- or 8-hour sleepers over the 16 years. Moreover, the apparently minor effect of short sleep as a possible cause of weight gain is further evident in the small but albeit highly statistically significant 0.9 kg greater weight of the 5-hour sleepers compared with those sleeping 8 hours, found at the start of the study, when presumably all had been sleeping in this manner for some years before then.

Three other recent, large prospective cohort studies are also noteworthy. The first [6] undertook a 5-year follow-up of 522 men and women. For those originally aged under 40 years, who habitually slept fewer than 5 hours, and compared with 6–7 hour sleepers, there was a 1.8 greater increase in BMI over this period. Comparison between 6–7 hour sleepers and those sleeping over 8 hours, found a 0.9 greater increase in BMI for these 'longer' sleepers. However, for those who were originally aged over 40 years, no such overall effects were found. A 1.8 greater BMI equates roughly to about 6 kg (presumably mostly fat) for the typical man, which is about 1.2 kg per year, here. It is roughly comparable in energy content from eating, each month, just one cheeseburger with French fries (approx. 1000 calories—and assuming an approximate 70 % conversion of this energy into fat).

The second of these prospective studies [7] monitored 31,447 men and 3770 women for a year. For both groups there was no change in BMI for those habitually sleeping 7–8 hours, and almost zero BMI change for each of the three male groups sleeping 5–6, 6–7, and 8–9 hours. However, for men sleeping outside the range 5–9 hours there were significant but slight BMI gains of 0.07, which amounts to about a 200 g increase in body weight. None of the female groups showed any changes.

Thirdly, a UK study [8] of 3619 men and 1422 women initially compared BMIs and waist circumferences of habitually 7-hour sleeping adults with those sleeping (by self-estimates): fewer than 5 hours, at 6, 8, and over 9 hours. The shortest sleeping group had a small but statistically significantly greater BMI of 0.82, and a larger waist circumference of 1.9 cm. However, the investigators concluded that these minor differences were not sufficient enough to presume that short sleep was of particular importance to these differences. A subsequent follow-up, some 4–5 years later, found no relationship between short sleep and BMI changes. More interesting, was the finding that within the shortest sleepers, 25 % of the men and 33 % of the women were depressed, compared with values ranging between 8 % and 14 % for both men and women for the other hourly sleep categories, including for those sleeping longer than 9 hours.

There have been other case-control studies further pointing to little real association between sleep and obesity, e.g. [9–11], including meta-analyses (see Sect. 3.5) that have combined the various findings. A substantial meta-analysis [12] concluded that a habitual sleep reduction of 1 hour per day below 7 hours is associated with a 0.35 increase in BMI, per year, which is only about 1 kg for the average (1.8 m) height man. Again, it is apparent, as with other reviews [13], that any significant weight differences between short and 'normal' sleepers are small, very slow to accrue, even after many years of sleeping in this manner. Moreover, there remains no sound explanation for how short sleep might be the cause of this very slow weight gain.

Obesity itself can create discomfort and disturbance during sleep, apart from causing obstructive sleep apnoea (Sect. 9.3). Moreover, obese people tend to report higher incidences of insomnia linked to chronic emotional stress [14], although there appears to be no obvious difference in self-reported sleep duration between those obese and non-obese individuals who are free of chronic stress [14]. That is, emotional stress seems to have a stronger relationship with reported sleep duration than BMI, to the extent that short sleep in obese individuals might mostly be a sign of emotional stress. Given that shortened sleep in the form of early morning awakening is one of the diagnostic criteria for depression, then a disproportionate number of short sleepers would be expected to be depressed, irrespective of obesity [15]. An association between obesity and psychiatric problems has also been described by others as, for example, in a survey [16] of 9125 respondents, obesity was linked to a 25 % greater incidence of mood and anxiety disorders compared with the non-obese. Indeed, outside the topic of sleep, there is a clear link between depression and obesity [17], as well as with 'comfort eating' [18], but as the weight gain in very short sleepers attributable to their sleep is generally slow to develop, then the extent to which excess comfort eating is to blame, here, must be small.

While acute sleep restriction to 4 or 5 hours a night for several nights in healthy lean adults [1–3] increases appetite and hunger, one must bear in mind that if food is freely available to sleep-deprived participants who have little else to do, as has also been reported for other experimental studies of this nature [18, 19], then participants might well eat or snack more readily. Although such findings have been used to explain obesity in habitually very short sleepers, the very slow weight gain in such sleepers contrasts with that of these sleep restricted participants, who eat at least 300 calories a day in excess of the extra energy needed just by being awake for longer [18, 19]. As we have seen, someone habitually sleeping only 5 hours a day could put on maybe up to 2 kg of fat over a year. Roughly speaking, if this is converted back into calories at 9 calories per gram of fat, which is about 50 calories a day, this is much less than that seen in these acute experiments. It suggests that the increased food consumption in these experimental studies further points to it being undertaken under unusual conditions. However, there is a twist to my line of thinking, here, as habitually short sleep might well alter not so much body weight itself, but the regulation of energy balance in more subtle and hitherto unforeseen ways, to be covered in Sect. 12.3, concerning Rapid Eye Movement (REM) sleep.

Finally, rather than assess obesity levels in terms of sleep duration, it would be worthwhile to reverse these same findings and present them not as BMI for different sleep durations, but as mean sleep durations for normal BMI, versus overweight 26–29, and 30–34 (grade 1 obesity). Few studies focusing on obesity and sleep seem to have done this, however, the Swiss study [20] I mentioned previously (Sect. 3.5), which concentrated on cardiovascular disease, happened also to divide their 2162 patients into those whose BMI was either greater than or equal to 25 or below 25. Average sleep durations differed by 3 minutes, being 402 and 399 minutes respectively, and it should be remembered that those sleep durations were determined by EEGs, not by self-estimates.

4.4   Metabolic Syndrome and Type 2 Diabetes

Issues concerning the acute, severe sleep restriction studies on healthy young adults that pointed to the development of the metabolic syndrome were described at the beginning of this chapter. However, and in contrast, there is little epidemiological evidence to show that healthy, habitually 6-hour sleepers are at any seriously greater risk for developing metabolic syndrome. For example in a study [21] of 1214 participants aged 30 to 54 years, of whom 268 had the syndrome, 18 % of the 7–8 hour sleepers had it compared with 24 % for 6–7 hour sleepers, 28 % for those sleeping fewer than 6 hours, and 24 % for the longer than 8-hour sleepers; all of which seem to be similarly high incidences, but with only a 6 % difference between 6 and 8 hour sleepers. In terms of inverting these findings from the perspective of those who are symptom free, the figures seem less persuasive, being between 72 % and 82 % for all sleep groups.

Yet, as the metabolic syndrome and type 2 diabetes have been seen as 'inflammatory responses' [22], it could be argued that inadequate sleep has an adverse effect on immunity; hence this response. However, it will be remembered from Sect. 3.7 that short sleep or sleep loss leads only to equivocal changes in human immune function, which are not necessarily detrimental but may simply indicate heightened immunological activity (cf. [23]), and that one should exclude the animal studies in these respects [24, 25].

Concerning type 2 diabetes, the great majority of 6-hour sleepers sleeping in this manner over many years, with undisturbed sleep, are still unlikely to develop diabetes. For example, in the 10-year Nurses Health Study, described earlier (Sect. 4.3), the incidence of diabetes in 6-hour sleepers was 3.2 % compared with 2.5 % for 7- and 8-hour sleepers [26], which might be construed as a worryingly 30 % greater relative incidence for the former group, but if we again look at those who are symptom free, at 96.8 % and 97.5 % respectively, this apparently greater risk is very small. By the way, for those sleeping fewer than 5 hours and over 9 hours the incidences of diabetes were 4.0 % and 4.2 % respectively.

Even when the incidence of diabetes is higher, as was found in another large, long-term prospective study [27] reporting a doubling of the onset of diabetes in those sleeping fewer than 6 hours, at an incidence of 10 %, compared with 5 % for 7-hour sleepers, the onset was associated with up to 14 years of sleeping in this manner, and still with 90 % of these shorter sleepers remaining asymptomatic. Again, it cannot be established to what extent short sleep itself was even 'a' cause, rather than 'the' cause.

Finally, whilst a recent meta-analysis [28] encompassing 10 different studies concluded that 'short sleepers' have a 30 % increased risk of developing diabetes, it is quite clear from the findings of the individual studies that were incorporated, that much of this assertion only really applies to those sleeping fewer than 5 hours.

4.5   Overview: Unlikely Bedfellows?

The evidence behind the apparent link between habitual short sleep, obesity, metabolic syndrome and diabetes in adults does not point to short sleep as having more than a minor effect at best, although for those habitually sleeping fewer than 5 hours, this outcome might be somewhat more likely. Besides, there are various problems underlying many of these findings. Remember, sleep estimates are usually confounded by 'time in bed' and daytime naps, whilst largely ignoring sleep quality. There are wide categorisations of 'short sleep' still leading to claims and advocacy (cf. [29]) that less than 7 hours' sleep is associated with obesity and related illnesses, which stem mostly from generalisations from 5-hour sleepers who comprise about 6 % of adults. Other evidence comes from more extreme and unrealistic acute sleep restriction studies in healthy non-obese young adults, where the extent of the accompanying sleepiness would have been of a far greater immediate danger had they been outside the laboratory than the extent of their increases in appetite and insulin resistance. By far the majority of obese people are not short sleepers and for those very short sleepers, excessive daytime sleepiness may well be of much greater concern than obesity, especially if they suffer from undiagnosed obstructive sleep apnoea syndrome (cf. Sect. 9.3).

In terms of greater clinical importance are the statistically significant epidemiological findings of a greater body weight gain in 5-hour sleepers. Even then, any such weight gains accumulate slowly over years; these are more easily redressed by a better diet and relatively short daily exercise exposures, contrasting with the huge accumulation of 'lost' sleep. No study has really compared both interventions, and there is little evidence supporting 'more sleep', alone, as an effective treatment for obesity and these related disorders. Impaired sleep quality and quantity are symptoms of many deeper underlying physical and psychological disorders, as can be obesity.

Advocating more sleep could again heighten the anxieties of those with insomnia who might otherwise worry about becoming fat or developing diabetes as a result of insufficient sleep, thus heightening their use of sleep aids including hypnotics in order to lengthen sleep and seemingly offset obesity. But such interventions are unlikely to increase sleep duration by more than 30 minutes. So why not use this time for a healthier brisk walk, instead?

Of course, it could still be countered that the accumulated yearly health risk associated with 'short sleep', albeit small, is still a serious issue from an epidemiological perspective and, statistically, for example, might even be comparable to the year-on-year increased risk of smokers developing cardiovascular disease. However, excluding excessive daytime sleepiness, my conclusion here is that, irrespective of any causal link between short sleep and these disorders having yet to be established, and that a considerable amount of accumulated 'lost' sleep is required before any such association is seen, any such risk must be weighed against the lack of therapeutic effectiveness of extending sleep versus the benefits of more worthwhile behavioural countermeasures, especially exercise and a weight-reducing diet. Moreover, this healthier regimen will often lead to improved sleep and reduced daytime sleepiness in those overweight or moderately obese [30].

In sum, it is argued that the presumed effects of short sleep on obesity are not of such critical, clinical importance when put into these more realistic contexts. Unfortunately, it is all too tempting for press releases and the media to exaggerate the outcomes from the many reputable studies which themselves exercise caution in the interpretation of their own findings (cf. [31]).

References

1. Knutson KL et al 2007 The metabolic consequences of sleep deprivation. *Sleep Med Rev* 11: 163–178.
2. Spiegel K et al 1999. Impact of sleep debt on metabolic and endocrine function. *Lancet* 354, 1435–1439.
3. Leproult R, Van Cauter E. 2010 Role of sleep and sleep loss in hormonal release and metabolism. *Endocrol Devel* 17, 11–21.
4. Flegal KM, Kit BK, Graubard BI. 2013. Association of all-cause mortality with overweight and obesity using standard body mass index categories: a systematic review and meta-analysis' *J Amer Med Assoc* 309:1681–1682.
5. Patel SR et al 2006. Association between reduced sleep and weight gain in women. *Amer J Epidemiol* 164, 947–954.
6. Hairston KG et al 2010 Sleep duration and five-year abdominal fat accumulation in a minority cohort: the IRAS family study. *Sleep* 33, 289–295.
7. Watanabe M et al 2010 Association of short sleep duration with weight gain and obesity at 1-year follow-up: a large-scale prospective study. *Sleep* 33, 161–167.
8. Stranges S et al 2008 Cross-sectional versus prospective associations of sleep duration with changes in relative weight and body fat distribution: the Whitehall II Study. *Amer J Epidemiol* 167, 321–329.
9. Lauderdale DS et al 2009 Cross-sectional and longitudinal associations between objectively measured sleep duration and body mass index: the CARDIA Sleep Study. *Amer J Epidemiol* 170, 805–813.

10. Anic GM et al 2010 Sleep duration and obesity in a population-based study. *Sleep Med* 11: 447–451.

11. Nielsen LS, Danielsen KV. 2010 Short sleep duration as a possible cause of obesity: critical analysis of the epidemiological evidence. *Obes Rev* 12:78–92.

12. Cappuccio FP, et al 2008 Meta-analysis of short sleep duration and obesity in children and adults. *Sleep*; 31: 519–626.

13. Magee L, Hale L. 2012 Longitudinal associations between sleep duration and subsequent weight gain: a systematic review. *Sleep Med Rev.* 16: 231–241.

14. Vgontzas AN 2008 Short sleep duration and obesity: the role of emotional stress and sleep disturbances. *Int J Obesity* (London) 32, 801–809.

15. Meiseninger C 2007 Sleep duration and sleep complaints and risk of myocardial infarction in middle aged men and women from the general population: the MONICA/KORA Augsburg cohort study. *Sleep* 30, 1121–1127.

16. Simon GE 2006 Association Between Obesity and Psychiatric Disorders in the US Adult Population. *Arch Gen Psychiat* 63, 824–830.

17. McIntyre RS 2006, Obesity in bipolar disorder and major depressive disorder: results from a national community health survey on mental health and well-being. *Canada J Psychiatr* 51, 274–280.

18. Dallman MF 2009 Stress-induced obesity and the emotional nervous system. *Trend Endocrin Metab* 21, 159–165.

19. Markwald RR 2013. Impact of insufficient sleep on total daily energy expenditure, food intake, and weight gain. *Proc Natl Acad Sci U S A.* 110:5695–5700.

20. Haba-Rubio J et al. 2015. Objective sleep structure and cardiovascular risk factors in the general population: the HypnoLaus study. *Sleep*, 38: 391–400.

21. Spaeth AM 2013 Effects of experimental sleep restriction on weight gain, caloric intake, and meal timing in healthy adults. *Sleep* 36:981–990.

22. Hall MH et al 2008 Self-reported sleep duration is associated with the metabolic syndrome in midlife adults. *Sleep* 31, 635–643.

23. Bryant PA et al 2004. Sick and tired: does sleep have a vital role in the immune system? *Nature Rev Immunol*, 457–467.

24. Rechtschaffen A et al 2002. Sleep deprivation in the rat: X. Integration and discussion of the findings -1989. *Sleep*; 25, 68–87.

25. Horne JA. 1988 *Why we sleep*. Oxford: University Press.

26. Ayas NT et al 2003. A prospective study of self-reported sleep duration and incident diabetes in women. *Diabetes Care* 26, 380–384.

27. Yagg HK et al. 2006. Sleep duration as a risk factor for the development of type 2 diabetes. *Diabetes Care* 29, 657–661.
28. Holliday EG et al 2013 Short sleep duration is associated with risk of future diabetes but not cardiovascular disease: a prospective study and meta-analysis. *PLoS One* 25;8(11):e82305.
29. Watson NF et al 2015. Recommended amount of sleep for a healthy adult: a joint consensus statement of the American Academy of Sleep Medicine and Sleep Research Society. *Sleep* 38: 843–844.
30. Verhoef SPM et al. 2013. Concomitant changes in sleep duration, body weight and body composition during weight loss and 3-mo weight maintenance. *Am J Clin Nutr*, 98: 25–31.
31. Sumner P et al 2014. The association between exaggeration in health related science news and academic press releases: retrospective observational study. *BMJ* Dec 9;349:g7015. doi: 10.1136/bmj.g7015.

5

Childhood and Adolescence

Sleep is but one of the many needs of children, and it is foolish to make it the scape-goat for all kinds of physical and mental evils as hygienists have so often done. It is possible that the quantity of sleep is less important than its quality, and that when disturbances of the latter occur they are more likely to be the effect of ill-health than its cause ... sleep cannot be accurately measured in units of time alone ...

Terman & Hocking 1913.

5.1   Kids: Too Little Sleep?

Much is being said about today's children not having enough sleep, often blamed on lax bedtimes, excessive evening TV, video-gaming, etc. *Plus ça change*—a hundred or so years ago things were just as bad, even worse, when excessive homework was the culprit. For example, in 1884 the British Medical Journal reported that a Dr Crichton-Browne had testified to Parliament that, "*I have encountered many lamentable instances of derangement of health, diseases of the brain, and even death resulting from enforced evening study in young children, with the nervous excitement it so often induces ... it implies a maximum of effort with a minimum result*".

© The Editor(s) (if applicable) and The Author(s) 2016
J. Horne, *Sleeplessness*, DOI 10.1007/978-3-319-30572-1_5

Albeit wise but ignored words, he remained persistent, as in 1908 [1] the now knighted Sir James Crichton-Browne, in his presidential address to the Child Study Society bemoaned that, "*the evil of insufficient sleep in children is widespread*". He was responding to the talk by Dr Alice Ravenhill who had just described her three-year-long investigation into the sleep of elementary schoolchildren. Ten thousand forms had been issued of which 6180 "*were properly filed up, and gave particulars as to 3500 boys and 2680 girls*". Having previously "*consulted the best authorities*" who had apparently advocated 13 hours' sleep for the younger group and 11 hours' for the older ones, she had calculated a sleep deficiency ranging from 2.75 to 3.25 hours, depending on the age. For example, for the 3–5 year group she found the average sleep obtained was 10.75 hours versus the recommended standard of 14 hours, and at 13 years the average was only 8 hours against the recommended 10.30 hours. Both of these actual findings are somewhat less than those of today, as will be seen. Nevertheless, Sir James went on to comment that this represented "*a loss equivalent to one night in four in the youngest children, and one night in five among those of intermediate ages*".

There are two more studies of note, appearing around the same time, from different countries. In 1907, a Dr L Bernhard published [2] a similar study on 6551 German children aged between 6 and 14 years. And in 1913 came the still renowned report from the USA by Drs Lewis Terman and Alice Hocking [3] on, 'The sleep of schoolchildren: its distribution according to age and its relation to physical and mental efficiency'.

Bernhard's findings point to children's bedtimes being later then than today, but with similar morning rising times. Further details of his findings are given in the table below, including those of Ravenhill and, more importantly, from the remarkably thorough and still unique study by Terman and Hocking, that I will now describe.

It was based on 2692 Californian children and, most importantly, avoided asking parents to complete the questions on behalf of their children, but rather asked the children themselves about their sleep, with the children having received very clear and impartial guidance from their teachers. It might be argued that younger children are not really able to do this, but the study was so well organised and, remember, it was a hundred years ago when reading and writing skills were as good as, and arguably better, age for age, than today. Nevertheless, since then, including the present day, I know of no other such discerning study on sleep involving children themselves. Teachers were given a 300 word instruction sheet on how to proceed. For example, on the day before the sleep records were to be collected and just before dismissal of school in the afternoon, teachers were to ask the pupils how many hours they liked to sleep. *"Tell them to look at the clock 'tonight' just as they go to bed and to write down on a piece of paper the exact time. (Make it clear that they are to make the record just as soon as they look at the clock.) Tell them also to look at the clock again as soon as they wake up next morning and to record the time on the same piece of paper ... bring it to school next day. Make no other request or announcement. Be especially careful to avoid giving any suggestion as to the amount of sleep you think children should have. Say nothing about windows."* Next day, as soon as school assembled, question sheets were distributed and the pupils were asked to answer all the questions they could and were not to try to answer those they were not sure about. Above all, teachers were asked to make clear *'that no one will be reproached for having forgotten to make the records or for inability to answer any of the questions. Pupils are not to be encouraged to guess'.*

These questions included: How long do you think it took you to go to sleep? Did anyone have to wake you? How many others slept in the same room and same bed? Did you sleep your usual amount last night? If not, was it more or less than usual? How much? How many hours per week do you work outside of school? At that time, much emphasis was placed on the need for children to get plenty of fresh air, and this is why there were also questions on the number of windows that were open in the night and how wide open they were.

As no differences in sleep durations were found between boys and girls, Terman and Hocking combined these findings. The table compares the fairly consistent findings, age for age, for these three studies, and I want to stay on this topic a little longer, as not only were there other pertinent comments made by Terman and Hocking at the time, but their findings also show that sleep for today's children has changed little since then, despite current beliefs about the inadequacy of our children's sleep. Moreover, their study has consistently been misreported as evidence claiming that adults in those days slept for longer than today, at around

9 hours. Clearly, this is wrong as their research was based on schoolchildren, not adults, with the oldest being 18 years.

Terman was an educational psychologist well known at the time for his development of IQ tests, and had a particular interest in children's ability at school. However, he and Hocking noticed, in their prescient report: *a lack of correlation we have found between school success and hours of sleep; namely, that large quantitative differences in sleep may be fully offset by qualitative differences. If this be true then sleep cannot be accurately measured in units of time alone ... It is possible that the margin of safety is so large that both body and mind will for many years withstand with apparent success a surprising deficiency of sleep ... If, as seems to be the case, our study offers evidence that the average hours of sleep secured by American children include a large margin of safety, we are not compelled to conceive of this average as representing in any sense an excess of sleep ...*

In comparing their own findings with those of Ravenhill and of Bernhard, Terman and Hocking noted that their (Terman and Hocking's) children slept for longer, and the investigators asked, "*Why this astonishing difference?*" and then gave three explanations. The first was with what they saw to be the most important, being the climate of California which allowed for "*a far greater amount of outdoor life than is possible (or at least customary) in Germany and England*". The second was more contentious as they argued that "*the home environment of our children is probably much superior to that of the children studied by Bernhard and Ravenhill. Their statistics were collected mostly in industrial cities, ours in the smaller and more comfortable cities in the best sections of the United States, where the extreme overcrowding and poverty so common in European industrial centers are hardly known*". More interesting is their noting that US schools began at 9 a.m. instead of the customary 8 a.m. found in most European countries at that time.

However, today, this latter situation has reversed as most schools in the USA now start much earlier, at around 7.30 a.m., often with children having to be 'bussed in' from long distances, necessitating their having to get up at 6 a.m., often earlier. Although this allows schools to end earlier in the day, around lunch time, many children are too sleepy at school to learn, which is why many well-known sleep scientists in the USA continue to call for later school start times, as it happens, like those we have in the UK, at around 8.30–9.00 a.m.

The recent impressive historical analysis, by Dr Lisa Matricciani and colleagues [4, 5] from the University of South Australia, of sleep trends in a total of 690,000 children aged 5–18 years, was based on reports over the last 100 years, and from 20 countries. She concluded that, on average, primary schoolchildren from these countries are sleeping, today, at only around 30 minutes less than they once did. For adolescents this fall is about 90 minutes. As one might expect, there are differences between countries, with children in Australia and the UK seeming to reverse this trend by sleeping about 1 hour longer than they did 100 years ago, whereas in mainland Europe, USA and Canada it is about 1 hour less, with no change for Scandinavia. This [4, 5] was a thorough study, utilising actual findings, unlike several other studies of this nature that often make repeated references to the same indirect sources, without consulting the original findings. That is, these other studies often cite those findings second- or even third-hand.

Clearly, for any age group there are large, natural variations in sleep duration, and the findings I have just described mostly concern averages. However, a closer look at an analysis [6] from the USA on changes in sleep duration among adolescents, from 1991 until 2012, is more revealing, as it focused on those who slept fewer than 7 hours. Over the 20 years, just over 272,000 adolescents in 3 age bands (13, 15 and 17 years), were each sampled once only. Two questions were asked, with the key one being, 'how often do you get at least 7 hours sleep?' Responses were on a 6-point scale from 'never' to 'every day'. The other question was rather vaguer, being 'how often do you get less sleep than you should?', also using the same 6-point scale. Responses for 'every day' or 'almost every day' were compared with 'sometimes', 'rarely' or 'never'. The overall percentage for those claiming fewer than 7 hours' sleep had risen by about 10 % over the 20 years, and those reporting 'less than you should', had risen by about 7 %. Although both changes are highly statistically significant, these are perhaps not so alarming in terms of actual percentages.

Of course, cultures vary considerably in attitudes and practices towards children's sleep, and an excellent account of this has come from Dr Oskar Jenni and colleagues [7] from the University of Zurich. For example,

Table 5.1 Historical comparisons of children's sleep from three studies and countries, Bernhard (Germany, 1907), Ravenhill (UK, 1908) and Terman and Hocking (USA, 1913)

Age in years	6–7	7–8	8–9	9–10	10–11	11–12	12–13	13–14	14–15	15–16	16–17	17–18
			Sleep in hours and minutes									
Bernhard	10.20	9.50	9.25	9.20	9.10	8.55	7.50	n/a	n/a	n/a	n/a	n/a
Ravenhill boys	10.30	10.30	9.30	9.15	9.15	8.45	8.15	8.30	n/a	n/a	n/a	n/a
Ravenhill girls	10.45	10.30	10.55	9.30	9.30	9.15	8.00	7.30	n/a	n/a	n/a	n/a
Terman & Hocking	11.14	10.41	10.42	10.13	9.56	10.0	9.36	9.31	9.06	8.54	8.30	8.46

in northern Europe and the USA today's children tend to have stricter bedtime routines and earlier bedtimes than those in southern Europe and Latin America, where there is more flexibility, often with children joining evening meals and other family gatherings, only to fall asleep at some point and be put to bed.

A recent survey of 11,000 UK children [8] has found that the average 6-year-old sleeps 11.3 hours, and for 10-year-olds it is 10.5 hours, which are very close to those found by Terman and Hocking, and longer than those of Bernhard and of Ravenhill (Table 5.1).

Before ending this historical account of sleep in children, it is worth remembering that so much of the guidance to new parents of today, given by various authorities, was so wisely described by the Victorians. Take for example, this advice aimed at parents of very young infants, provided by the British Medical Journal in 1869 [9], albeit rather austerely written, with a hint of irony, but to the point and still appropriate today. In his article 'On Sleeplessness in Infants' Dr Eustace Smith wrote:

By far the most common cause of restlessness at night is injudicious feeding, the child being stuffed with food, which, although not necessarily in itself injurious is yet ill-adapted to the nourishment of the particular infant to whom it is given … Cold feet are not an infrequent cause of wakefulness in infants … The feet in infants should be always carefully warmed before the children are out to bed … Children who are too much petted and indulged, easily contract habits which are sources of great annoyance, not only to themselves, but also to those through whose uncalculating tenderness the habit has been acquired. Thus in little children little attention should be paid to cries excited by other causes other than actual suffering or discomfort. Cries from wilfulness or fretfulness should be entirely disregarded ... the mother may satisfy herself that his cries are not produced by cold feet or colicky pains ... and he should be left in his cot to cry himself asleep. If not, and he be taken up and hushed in the arms of his mother, the probabilities are very strongly in favour of his waking and crying at about the same hour on the succeeding night, and requiring to be pacified by the same means. A habit is thus gradually acquired, which it is very difficult afterwards to overcome. Infants accustomed to be suckled at frequent intervals during the night are also exceedingly restless. This is a practice which cannot be too strongly condemned. Children should be accustomed early to take no food during the night. A very young infant, who has been suckled immediately before the mother retires to rest will do well until five or six o'clock on the following morning without a further supply of nourishment. He is easily made to understand that this is a rule which cannot be infringed, and will wake and sleep again without disturbance if he knows it is useless to complain.

5.2 Growth

Sleep is opportune for growth in children, and for at least two associated reasons. Levels of growth hormone and other growth promoting hormones are more evident in their sleep than in wakefulness, partly because excessive physical activity during wakefulness will delay any growth until a fairly prolonged rest occurs, as with sleep. However, for the child merely lying resting at night, but awake instead of sleep, this sleep-related growth hormone surge is suppressed (but not entirely), and thus actual growth will probably be less apparent, although this remains poorly explored. Nevertheless, there is no evidence pointing to any association between sleep duration and actual growth in children [10]. For example, longer sleepers are not taller. Most short children remain short and most tall children remain tall as they become older and, similarly, shorter and longer sleepers tend to remain like this within their age group as they become older [10]. Both these characteristics, height and sleep, are largely 'phenotypic' being environmentally and genetically determined, and independent of each other [10]. On the other hand, stress in a child, whether it be physical, medical or psychological, will inhibit growth, interfere with growth hormone release especially at night, and also cause sleep disturbance (rather than shorter sleep).

Certainly in the western world, and irrespective of sleep, children are taller and healthier today than just a few generations ago, thanks to better nutrition, sanitation, medicines, vaccinations, etc. Although childhood obesity is becoming an issue, this really relates to diet and exercise, rather than to sleep (see Sect. 5.3).

Interestingly, if a child's height is measured at bedtime and again the next morning, they will be taller by over half a centimetre depending on age, which might suggest a remarkable degree of overnight growth. But, by the following bedtime they would have shrunk back again. It is the lying down, not sleep itself that allows the cartilage found between the vertebrae (intervertebral discs) and at the ends of leg bones ('epiphyses'), to absorb water and expand by a minute amount, which together will increase height, only to become compressed back to normal when standing up and moving about. Likewise, this happens with the arms, as they become a little longer, then shorter in the same manner. This effect also applies to the intervertebral discs of adults (no epiphyses in adults), where this temporary height difference can be a centimetre or more.

5.3   Obesity

Like those for adults, epidemiological studies on children are reporting statistically significant correlations between short sleep and obesity, often seen to be part of an 'obesity epidemic', and linked to claims about children sleeping fewer hours today, although this is not borne out to any great extent, as I have pointed out. Again, this significant link is of questionable clinical significance, for several reasons, and largely because of similar methodological problems I described for adults (Chap. 3). In these studies on children, to assess obesity, estimates of children's sleep durations are usually based on parental responses to a single question, and with few studies defining 'sleep' versus 'time in bed'. Moreover, school days versus weekends/holidays are often overlooked. And, as before, any such weight gains in shorter sleepers are probably accumulated over a year or so of sleeping like this; that is, after some hundreds of hours of apparently 'less sleep', there are only small increases in BMI for those shorter sleepers. By the way, BMI as an index of child obesity is itself a debatable topic [11]. Finally, these studies tend to split sleepers into those children who sleep either more or less than (usually) 10 hours a night to those sleeping far below this threshold, who might indeed be at a greater risk of obesity.

Several case-control studies, e.g. [12–14], have reported the prevalence of obesity in those children sleeping fewer than 10 hours to be double that for those sleeping longer. But there is another perspective, as one report [12], also finding a doubling of the proportion of shorter sleepers who were obese (7.7 %) compared with (3.6 %) for the longer sleepers, is not so impressive if one inverts this finding. That is, the remaining 92.3 % versus 96.4 % were of normal weight. Similarly, whilst a later report [13] found that 5.4 % of short sleepers were obese, which was double for those sleeping longer than 10 hours (2.8 %), this difference is again small when seen from the alternative perspective. In another study [14] finding a significant negative correlation between sleep duration and body weight in boys, sleep duration only accounted for 10 % of the total effect on weight (compared with other factors), which was not significant for girls.

There have been many prospective cohort studies. For example in one well-known investigation [15], 785 children (equal numbers of boys and girls) were monitored from ages 9 to 12 years, and a significant link was found between short sleep and their becoming overweight. Also assessed were: the 'level of chaos at home', 'quality of the home environment' and 'lax-parenting'. By 12 years, 17.7 % of these children were overweight, and their sleep duration averaged 8.8 hours, which was significantly shorter than the 9.02 hours for normal weight children. However, this difference was only about 14 minutes, including a 7 minute average later bedtime for those who were overweight. Nevertheless, the investigators extrapolated these findings to propose that for every extra hour of sleep at age 9, children were 40 % less likely to be overweight by the age of 12.

The impressively large 'Avon' prospective study [16] of 7758 UK children (equal numbers of boys and girls) monitored from birth and subsequently assessed at 8 years of age found, from using BMIs, that 9.2 % of the boys and 8.1 % of the girls were obese. When these BMIs were compared with sleep durations previously obtained at age 3 years, 8 factors were found to be associated with the risk of subsequent obesity, including: parental obesity, watching television for more than 8 hours per week, and short (less than 10.5 hours) sleep. Even so, over the 5 years, 89.7 % of these short sleepers had normal BMIs, compared with 93.2 % for those sleeping over 12 hours. But, note, I have inverted these findings from the reported 10.3 % and 6.7 % respectively, which showed a significant difference.

Similarly small but significantly lesser amounts of habitual sleep in overweight children were described in another prospective study [17] monitoring children from birth to 9.5 years of age. Five independent risk factors were identified: parent overweight, child temperament, low parental concern about child weight, food tantrums and daily sleep at age 3–5 years. Daily sleep duration at this earlier age was negatively related to becoming overweight, and for those who did become fatter, they slept about 30 fewer minutes than those of normal weight. However, 25 minutes of this comprised shorter daytime sleep (unclear why), with only a 5 minute difference in night sleep. The strongest factor relating to becoming overweight, here, was parental BMI.

There are many more studies of this nature, cf. [18], and the ones I have described are quite typical. I should emphasise that I am not critical of these studies or their findings, but with the implications, which I have seen from a different perspective. That is, sleep has a much smaller impact on body weight in children than is often claimed. The complexities involved with unravelling any link between sleep and obesity in children is reflected by a discerning study from Japan [19], looking at lifestyle, social characteristics and obesity in 9674 Japanese children aged 3 years old. Of those sleeping less than 10 hours, 29 % were obese. Corrections for sex and various social variables showed the following to be related to obesity: irregular snacking; physical inactivity; household family including grandparents; mother as main caregiver but in full-time employment; attending a nursery; shorter sleeping hours (which seemed to indicate fewer hours allowed for the child to sleep). Another study [20] of 1676 mother-infant pairs, found that during the first 2 years of life, maternal depression, age at introduction of solids, attendance at child care facilities outside the home, being black, Hispanic or Asian, all contributed to shorter sleep in these infants.

Some meta-analyses have been quite forthright in arguing for the benefits of longer sleep for offsetting obesity in children, for example [21], "*the prevalence of childhood obesity may be decreased by increasing sleep duration independent of other risk factors*" (p. 272), which seems to be overstated, especially as these conclusions were based on standardised sleep durations and heavily reliant on statistically significant pooled odds ratios. Besides, there are also studies reporting short sleep duration having no effect on body weight in children, as found by another large prospective study [22] on sleep and BMI in about 3800 children monitored from birth until 7 years, which concluded that sleep duration did not predict obesity at any period during development. The detailed US National Survey of Children's Health [23] conducted in 2003, on 81,390 children aged between 6 and 17 years, reported no relationship between sleep duration and BMI after socio-demographic variables were included, with the authors concluding "*that the role of insufficient sleep in the childhood obesity epidemic remains unproven*" (p. 153).

In fact there is indeed little or no evidence that by extending the sleep of short-sleeping, overweight children, it will prevent or reverse any further increase in body fat. Even early 'prophylactic' sleep interventions with poor sleeping infants do not reduce the incidence of their becoming overweight [24]. Thus, to repeat my well-worn message, better dietary management coupled with more physical exercise are much more likely to help maintain normal body weight in children, as well as having other health benefits.

5.4   Of Greater Concern

Unfortunately, obesity in children can also lead to their having obstructive sleep apnoea (OSA, see Sect. 9.3), with one of the earliest accounts given by Charles Dickens in his *Pickwick Papers*, of Joe, the 'fat boy': "*The object that presented itself to the eyes of the astonished clerk, was a boy—a wonderfully fat boy—habited as a serving lad, standing upright on the mat, with his eyes closed as if in sleep … 'Sleep!' said the old gentleman, 'he's always asleep. Goes on errands fast asleep, and snores as he waits at table.' 'How very odd!' said Mr. Pickwick."*

Another problem for young children having persistently poor sleep is that they may not seem particularly sleepy, and rather than obesity, of greater concern are behavioural problems such as irritability, impatience, overactivity, novelty seeking, a need for constant stimulation and inability to concentrate, all of which resemble mild attention deficit hyperactivity disorder (ADHD). Treatment, here, should focus on rectifying the poor sleep. However, I must emphasise that lack of sleep is not the cause of more serious ADHD even though such children do have disturbed sleep. Nevertheless, some 20 % of children with the milder, apparent symptoms of ADHD can have a sleep-related breathing disorder. They are usually not obese, but are more likely to have enlarged tonsils, chronic throat infections, nose congestion and hay fever, all causing them to 'snuffle and snore' excessively at night, to the extent that they have OSA and severely disturbed sleep. For those with enlarged tonsils, a tonsillectomy can be the most appropriate treatment [25].

5.5   Late Nights

Adolescence is not only a time of physical growth but is when the cortex and its associated brain structures undergo 'rewiring' for adulthood, which affects behaviour in various ways, including emotions. As sleep is the only time when the cortex can go 'offline' to any extent, to recover from its waking workload and undertake adjustments, including this rewiring, then sleep for adolescents is particularly important.

Adolescence has almost always brought greater freedom from parental control, especially in the late evening when, nowadays, the young people are enlivened with the advent of electronic media, texting, and the accompanying 'social pressures' to keep online and up-to-date with one's peers. This excitement can delay sleep, as can the effect of evening bright light, particularly blue-tinged light (see Sect. 7.1) from TVs, computer screens and the like, which have a more direct action in delaying the body clock and its accompanying nocturnal melatonin surge. Thus, sleepiness is suppressed at their otherwise usual bedtime. Then there is the increasing tendency for teenagers to use caffeinated drinks in the evening [26] as happens especially with schoolchildren in the USA, where most also have in their bedroom a TV, mobile phone and a computer. In fact, having three or more technology items in the bedroom is [26] associated with 45 fewer minutes of sleep, compared with those children without such bedroom items. However, attempting to separate these young adults from their electronic paraphernalia at night is easier said than done, and I'm reminded by the view so eloquently put by Quentin Crisp: "*The young always have the same problem – how to rebel and conform at the same time. They have now solved this by defying their parents and copying one another.*"

Thus, for one reason or another teenagers become more 'evening types' and in order to maintain even 8 hours' sleep they would need to wake up later. But, of course, on schooldays they cannot do this, particularly in countries where schools begin at around 7.30 a.m. or even earlier, as in the USA. Inevitably, despite the parents' best but fruitless intentions for that earlier bedtime, sleep can be inadequate and there is sleepiness in class which impairs learning [27]. However, thanks to lying-in during weekends and school vacations, there is usually much opportunity for quick recovery. Although studies from several countries point to impaired school performance in these respects, it is unclear whether sleep loss itself is always the real issue, rather than due to emotional and related causes leading to inadequate sleep, and not simply overcome by earlier bedtimes, for example. Thus, after excluding TV viewing, depression, diet, lack of exercise and poor parental education, even this apparent effect of lack of sleep on school performance disappears or, at best, is bidirectional, with complex interactions between all these factors [27].

To accommodate these changes in sleep patterns in adolescence, some schools in the UK have adopted even later start times for older teens in an attempt to provide for more sleep, despite what many parents regard as already reasonable school start times (typically 8.30–9.00 a.m.) Initially, at least, and with eager support from pupils and teachers alike, there have been improvements to scholastic performance, here, which might have little to do with sleep itself, but result from a 'placebo effect' due to general enthusiasm. Moreover, bedtimes might just become later, pro rata. However, a proper controlled study is almost impossible in practical terms, with classes having to be randomly split between normal and later start times, and with teachers who can enthuse to the same extent about either start time. Besides, there are complications with different transportation times to and from school, especially for families where younger siblings are involved, and when working parents are constrained time-wise. Other difficulties might well include after-school sports having to be delayed, especially into darkness during winter months.

Finally, returning to obesity and sleep, but in adolescents, there is little evidence that habitually short sleep by itself, even if it persisted throughout school periods and vacations, would be associated with obesity to any remarkable extent, here. The National Longitudinal Study of Adolescent Health, undertaken in the USA, covering many aspects of health in 12–18 year olds, included over 13,000 adolescents who were also asked about their sleep duration. Their overall average age was almost 16 years, with an average sleep duration of 7.9 hours, and 10.6 % were obese. However, when non-sleep factors were taken into consideration, such as depression, watching too much TV, physical inactivity, skipping breakfast and eating fast food for more than 2 days per week, there was no association between sleep duration and obesity [27]. Those who were depressed were twice as likely to be obese, and those who watched more than 2 hours of TV per day were 37 % more liable to be so. A later reanalysis of these findings [28] but in a much smaller sample, found that an even greater link with obesity was the consumption of caffeinated drinks, with the authors concluding: "*The complex relationships between caffeine intake and the use of technology with shortened periods of sleep and increased BMI need further study*" (p. 286).

References

1. Crichton-Browne J 1908 Presidential address to the child study society. *Nature* Vol 79 p 28.
2. Bernhard L 1907 *Beitr Kin-derf Heilerziehung* Vol 39 issue 5 Pp5–13.
3. Terman L, Hocking A 1913 The sleep of schoolchildren: its distribution according to age and its relation to physical and mental efficiency'. *J Educ Psychol* 4:138–47 M.

4. Matricciani L et al 2011 A review of evidence for the claim that children are sleeping less than in the past. *Sleep* 34:651–659.

5. Matricciani L et al 2012 In search of lost sleep: secular trends in the sleep time of school-aged children and adolescents *Sleep Med Rev.* 16:203–211.

6. Keyes KM et al 2015 The great sleep recession: changes in sleep duration among US adolescents 1991–2012 *Pediatrics*, 135: in press.

7. Jenni OG, O'Connor BB. 2005 Children's sleep: an interplay between culture and biology. *Pediatrics.* 115: (Suppl 1):204–216.

8. Blair PS et al 2012 Childhood sleep duration and associated demographic characteristics in an english cohort. *Sleep.* 35:353–360.

9. Smith E 1869 On sleeplessness in infants *Br Med J* Aug 28 p236.

10. Jenni OG et al 2007 Sleep duration from ages 1 to 10 years: variability and stability in comparison with growth *Pediatrics.* 120:e769–e776.

11. Himes JH 2009 Challenges of accurately measuring and using BMI and other indicators of obesity in children. *Pediatrics* 124 Suppl 1 S3–S22.

12. Locard E et al 1992. Risk factors in obesity in a five year old population. Parental versus environmental factors. *Int J Obesity* 16: 721–729.

13. Von Kries R et al 2002. Reduced risk for overweight in 5 and 6-y-old children by duration of sleep – a cross sectional study. *Int J Obesity* 26: 710–716.

14. Chaput J-P et al 2006. Relationship between short sleeping hours and childhood overweight/obesity: results from the 'Quebec en Forme' Project. *Int J Obesity* 30: 1080–1085.

15. Lumeng J et al 2007 Shorter sleep duration is associated with increased risk of being overweight at ages 9 to 12 years. *Pediatrics* 120: 1020–1029.

16. Reilly JJ et al 2005 Early life risk factors for obesity in childhood: cohort study. *Br Med J* 330: 1357–1363.

17. Agras WS et al 2004 Risk factors for childhood overweight: a prospective study from birth to 9.5 years. *J Pediat.* 145: 20–25.

18. Horne J. 2011 Obesity and short sleep: unlikely bedfellows. *Obes Rev* 12: e84–e94.

19. Kagamimori S 1999 The relationship between lifestyle, social characteristics and obesity in 3-year-old Japanese children. *Child Care Health Devel.* 25: 235–247.

20. Nevarez MD et al 2010 Associations of early life risk factors with infant sleep duration. Acta Pediatr 10:187–193.

21. Chen X et al 2008 Is sleep duration associated with childhood obesity? A systematic review and meta-analysis. *Obesity.* 16: 265–274.

22. Hiscock H et al 2011 Sleep duration and body mass index in 0-7 year olds. *Arch Dis Child* 96: 735–739.

23. Hassan F et al 2011 No independent association between insufficient sleep and childhood obesity in the National Survey of Children's Health. *J Clin Sleep Med.* 7:153–157.

24. Wake M et al 2011 Does an intervention that improves infant sleep also improve overweight at age 6? Follow-up of a randomised trial. *Arch Dis Child* 96:526–532.

25. Sedky K et al 2014 Attention deficit hyperactivity disorder and sleep disordered breathing in pediatric populations: a meta-analysis *Sleep Med Rev.* 18:349–56.

26. Calamaro CJ et al 2012 Wired at a young age: the effect of caffeine and technology on sleep duration and body mass index in school-aged children. *J Pediatric Health Care* 26:276–282.

27. Shochat T et al 2014. Functional consequences of inadequate sleep in adolescents: a systematic review *Sleep Med Rev.* 18:75–87.

28. Calamaro CJ et al 2010 Shortened sleep duration does not predict obesity in adolescents *J Sleep Res* 19:559–556.

6

When Is Enough, Enough?

Most people oversleep 100 per cent, because they like it. That extra 100 per cent makes them unhealthy and inefficient. The person who sleeps eight or ten hours a night is never fully asleep and never fully awake—they have only different degrees of doze through the twenty-four hours. ... For myself I never found need of more than four or five hours' sleep in the twenty-four. I never dream. It's real sleep. When by chance I have taken more I wake dull and indolent. We are always hearing people talk about 'loss of sleep' as a calamity. They better call it loss of time, vitality and opportunities. Just to satisfy my curiosity I have gone through files of the British Medical Journal and could not find a single case reported of anybody being hurt by loss of sleep. Insomnia is different entirely— but some people think they have insomnia if they can sleep only ten hours every night.

Thomas Edison 1888

6.1   Priorities

Sleep still remains a vulnerable state to be in, less so today, but nevertheless its most important functions will have priority, appearing soon after sleep onset. Sleep is by the brain, primarily for the recovery of the cerebral cor-

© The Editor(s) (if applicable) and The Author(s) 2016
J. Horne, *Sleeplessness*, DOI 10.1007/978-3-319-30572-1_6

tex from the effects of prior wakefulness (see Sect. 10.1), and it seems that this recovery is largely reflected by the deepest and most unconscious form of sleep, 'slow wave sleep' (SWS), mentioned in earlier chapters. To recap, SWS is characterised in the EEG by high amplitude 'delta' (0.5–3.5 Hz) EEG waves, with the lesser and more intense form of SWS known as Stages 3 and 4 sleep respectively. A newer convention has renamed SWS as 'S3' sleep, but to avoid confusion I will keep to 'SWS', which typically appears during normal sleep as three diminishing bouts, separated by periods of REM sleep (REM) and lighter (Stages 1 and 2) non-REM sleep (see Sect. 10.5). Unlike SWS, successive periods of REM become longer and more intense. Whereas SWS depends largely on the duration of prior wakefulness, as will be seen shortly, REM seems, particularly, to be preparing us for oncoming wakefulness, and I will be arguing in Chap. 12, that REM can even act as a substitute for wakefulness. The typical course of these sleep stages is shown in the 'hypnogram' in Fig. 6.1.

Many studies dating back to the 1960s, cf. [1], have clearly shown this primacy of SWS, which is retained during sleep restriction and mostly recovered following total sleep deprivation, to a far greater extent than other sleep stages, including REM, cf.[1]. That is, much of the sleep lost during sleep deprivation is not recovered as it is the quality of this recovery sleep which is most important [2]. The next section describes this recovery process from the perspective of the 'two process model'.

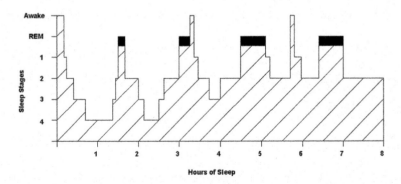

Fig. 6.1 Hypnogram showing the distribution of sleep stages over a typical night—note the 90-minute cycling and predominance of SWS at the beginning and REM at the end of sleep, respectively

However, the many findings that this lost sleep is actually lost have been questioned, because when sleep-deprived people are confined to bed for 24 hours following a night of total sleep loss, for example, and allowed to sleep ad lib, then seemingly much of the total lost sleep seems to be recovered. But I argue that this extra sleep largely falls into the category of a 'confinement-related surplus of sleep', to be covered shortly.

6.2   The End of Sleep

The timing of sleep as well as the daily rhythm of alertness are heavily influenced by the 24-hour circadian rhythm ('body clock'). Changes to body temperature as well as to alertness reflect the progress of this clock, with rises typically beginning about 5–6 a.m., usually coinciding with about 6 hours of sleep, increasing soon after normal morning wake-up time, with a levelling off, typically followed by a variable 'dip' around mid-afternoon. A final rise to an evening peak at around 7–9 p.m. is followed by a fall up to bedtime and beyond, until the daily circadian trough, at around 4 a.m., which is most apparent if and when one remains awake at this time. Whereas these 24 hour changes with alertness are relatively large, those of body temperature are fairly small—being about 0.7 °C from peak to trough. For the body as a whole, such a daily change in its 'core' temperature has little impact, whereas for the brain its temperature has to be so finely controlled, to the extent that even this small difference can noticeably affect its functions. Of course, people differ somewhat in these daily timings, as in 'larks and owls', which is the topic for Sect. 7.3.

The morning circadian rise acts as a natural sleep terminator. The interaction between sleep and the circadian clock is illustrated by the well-known 'two process model' [3], seen in Fig. 6.2. 'Process S' is a sleep pressure that builds up during wakefulness and discharges during sleep (seen as the hatched portions) with its declining intensity reflected mostly by SWS. 'Process C' (for 'circadian') continues almost relentlessly, regardless of sleep, facilitating sleep onset at night, and seen by the fall in body temperature and alertness at this time. The morning rise in Process C, with its braking effect on sleep, is particularly noticeable in those people having a regular morning wake-up time who, after a late night, are likely

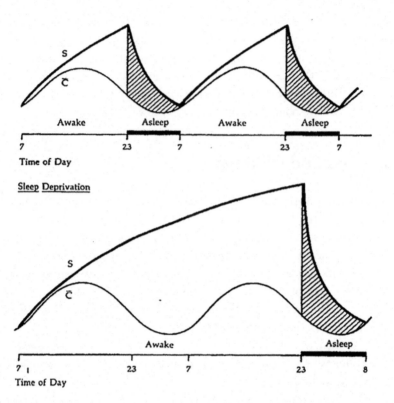

Fig. 6.2 The interaction of sleep pressure ('Process S') with the circadian rhythm ('Process C'), as in the 'two process model'. Upper figure—for a normal night. Lower figure—on a recovery night following a night of sleep loss. Note how the morning circadian rise acts as a sleep terminator—see text for details

to wake up still at this same time. The interactions between these two processes can be seen in the upper half of the figure, with the lower half illustrating what happens during a sleepless night, with the further, progressive build-up of Process S. Here, due to sleep pressure still remaining to a greater extent than usual at the normal wake-up time, there is some delay in this waking, with sleep continuing for a while, until the progressive morning rise of Process C overcomes Process S.

The model again reflects how, in terms of sleep duration, only a portion of lost sleep is recovered, with this mostly being SWS (Process S), when its greatest intensity is during the earlier part of this sleep. Although there might well be some more Process S (SWS) recovery the next night, usually necessitating an earlier bedtime, the normal morning awakening remains.

Having woken up at the circadian termination point, we can override it to some extent by a conscious decision to return to sleep as in a lie-in. However, the extent to which this latter sleep is 'refreshing' can be limited owing to the conflicting, continuing circadian rise, and sleeping 'out of phase' with the body clock. If this latter sleep is too extensive then it causes 'post sleep inertia', a form of temporary jet lag, typically experienced by night-shift workers when sleeping the following morning (see Sect. 7.5).

6.3 'Oversleep'

Some years before our better understanding of the interactions between sleep and the circadian rhythm, as reflected by the two process model, Dr Eugene Aserinsky, a pioneer in sleep research demonstrated that sleep reaches a satiation point after 7 hours of night sleep, and that further sleep was 'surplus to requirements'. In two unique studies [4, 5] he also showed that beyond this point REM becomes more intense, as if it had to do so in order to maintain this extra sleep. In these studies, he required healthy non-sleep-deprived volunteers to remain in bed, in quiet and darkened rooms for either 30 or 54 hours. They were encouraged to sleep as much as they could, which summated to averages of 20 and 32 hours sleep respectively. Most of this sleep was at night, with intermittent naps during the daytime. Although it could be argued that they must have had hidden 'sleep debt' and were merely making up for prior sleep loss (which Aserinsky denied), it is more likely they just slept beyond any real need. An important point I must add of my own is that, presumably, his participants would have been sleepy just before having these seemingly surplus sleeps, which also suggests that at least some of our sleepiness is 'situational and incidental' (more about this in Chap. 8).

Several less imposing studies have been undertaken with normal sleepers to see if similarly longer sleep improves waking alertness. One of the largest [6], involving 24 healthy volunteers who usually slept well, for 7–8 hours a night, encouraged them to sleep up to 10 hours per night for 6 nights. Prior to the extended sleep, half of them had initial MSLT latencies (i.e. propensity to sleep—see Sect. 1.6) of less than 6 minutes, indicating to the investigators that they had excessive daytime sleepiness, and were thus deemed to be 'sleepy' individuals. The others had much longer MSLT latencies, greater than 16 minutes, and were described as 'alert' individuals. Surprisingly, and following the extended sleep, the sleepy group only increased their MSLT scores by about 4 minutes, compared with 2–3 minutes for the 'alert' group. Reaction time testing showed no significant differences between the two groups before or after sleep extension. The rather puzzled authors concluded that, "*the performance results did not support the hypothesis of a differential improvement of sleepy versus alert subjects*".

We [7] found in our own study of 14 nights of similarly extended sleep in 8 healthy participants, who were monitored whilst sleeping in their own beds for up to 10 hours each night instead of their usual 8 hours, that they averaged an extra hour of sleep per night throughout the 2 weeks. There was no significant increase in daytime alertness (except for a minor reduction in the 'afternoon dip'), especially when they were tested on a variety of very sensitive psychological performance tests. In fact, there is little or no evidence from any sleep extension study, whether it be short or long term, that people who feel quite alert during the day, but nevertheless are able to extend their night sleep, have a greater ease of morning awakening, or feel more refreshed on arising, or are more alert throughout the day, cf. [8].

Similarly, mammals in zoos and laboratories, isolated from their natural habitat, safe from predators, well fed with no need to hunt for food, and relieved of the natural waking demands on their time, sleep for much longer than in their natural state. This cannot indicate that similar animals in the wild are habitually sleep deprived and are suffering perpetual sleep debt. Neither is there evidence pointing to these confined animals being more alert and vigorous in 'having had more sleep'—quite the opposite. Nor can it be shown that captivity creates a greater actual sleep need rather than just a sleep 'opportunity'. Thus they seem to be sleeping well in excess of any real need. Sheep in pens, horses in stables and cows in barns sleep much more than when in open fields, and pet cats sleep extensively compared with feral cats [1]. More fascinating is the three-toed sloth, which is one of the oddest and slowest of mammals, living upside down high in tropical rain forests. Renowned for their sleepiness, as seen in zoos, they sleep for around 16 hours a day, yet in their natural, wild state they sleep fewer than 10 hours daily, as was recently discovered [9] when their sleep was recorded, in the jungle, by utilising miniature EEG recorders attached to their heads. Do these animals forgo six hours daily sleep in the wild, making them so sleepy and the reason for their slowness? Or, given that they are no more alert or vigorous in the zoo, maybe they just sleep to excess, in confinement?

In sum, these findings again support there being a 'flexible' region towards the end of our normal, healthy nighttime sleep, which is beyond any real biological need.

6.4   'Social Jet Lag'

Sleeping for longer on vacations and at weekends is often an enjoyable indulgence, as well as including any recovery from sleep loss from previous days. For example, a large study [10] asking 1,500 respondents why they slept longer at weekends, found 'pleasure' to be the more likely answer rather than the alternative of 'making up for lost sleep'. Besides, a recent telephone survey by the US National Sleep Foundation [11] found that the extra sleep taken on Saturday and Sunday nights, when combined, only averaged a total of 72 minutes, suggesting either that sleep loss on weekdays was not profound, or that if this loss was greater, then only a portion of it was recovered, for whatever reasons.

Social jet lag is a recent, albeit attractive concept, largely advocated by Professor Till Roenneberg and colleagues from the University of Munich [12, 13]. They argue that for most of us, daily commitments, such as school and work hours, interfere with individual preferences in the timing of sleep, as determined by one's circadian clock, and that our sleep on 'work-free days' reflects our natural state. This discrepancy between social and biological time, that is, the mismatch between our internal clock and the realities of our daily schedules, is called 'social jet lag'. One's social jet lag can be calculated by taking the difference between the number of hours of sleep obtained on an average working weeknight (especially if woken by an alarm clock) from the number of hours of sleep without an alarm when one can sleep on until a spontaneous awakening. Thus, an apparent sleep debt can accumulate on workdays, with sleep recovered somewhat on the free days, with those of us who are evening types ('owls'—see Sect. 7.3) apparently showing the largest social jet lag and greater sleep debt, owing to later bedtimes.

In several respects sleep debt and social jet lag are synonymous, especially as not all of the lost sleep in weekdays is seen by Roenneberg to be recovered on work-free days and can lead to chronic sleep loss. Advocates of social jet lag recommend that work schedules should be adapted to one's own 'chronotype' (degree of 'morningness–eveningness'—see Sect. 7.3) whenever possible, and that we should make better use of daylight, as well as utilise daylight saving time to greater effect, especially as artificial light apparently weakens the more powerful effects of daylight on the body clock. Moreover, as social jet lag is most acute in adolescents, schools ought to start later, as already mentioned (Sect. 5.5).

Roenneberg has argued [12] that for adults between the ages of about 25 and 60 years, social jet lag has worsened somewhat over recent years, as sleep duration during workdays has become shorter, by around 30 minutes, whereas sleep on free days has lengthened by about 15 minutes. That is, on average, he finds that people sleep for about 7 hours on workdays and for about 45 minutes longer on free days. However, this is not a large difference, given that this extra sleep is also seen to contain recovery from the prior week's sleep loss.

Social jet lag is also associated with obesity [13], as there is a significant correlation between the extent of social jet lag and degree of being overweight or obese: the greater the social jet lag the more likely the obesity. But when compared with other links for being overweight (e.g., age, sex, socio-economic status, etc.) social jet lag only accounts for 8 % of all these variables [13]. In fact, actual obesity is only apparent, for whatever reasons, in people with a social jet lag greater than 3 hours [13]. That is, sleep is apparently 3 hours shorter on workdays, which is a large amount, and suggests that this group comprises a relatively high proportion of

5-hour weekday sleepers which, for most people, is clearly inadequate sleep (see Sect. 2.1).

Although social jet lag is an intriguing concept, I believe our sleep to be more flexible than social jet lag proponents imply, to the extent that any chronic sleep loss is not as severe as has been suggested. Also, this concept assumes that all sleep is equal in value in terms of recovery. For example, that the first hour of sleep is as important as the last hour, which is not the case. So, by measuring the timing of sleep on both work- and work-free days by taking the midpoint of sleep, as is also done when calculating social jet lag, this overlooks these qualitative changes during the course of sleep—that these halves are 'equipotent'. For example, with someone sleeping from midnight until 8 a.m. the sleep midpoint is arithmetically at 4 a.m., whereas in terms of sleep intensity and recovery, the 'biological midpoint' is earlier, more likely at 3 a.m.

6.5 More or Less

Several studies focusing on the sleepiness aspect of sleep need, systematically restrict normal sleep in healthy individuals, by one or more hours over several successive days. The often cited and impressive such study by Dr Hans van Dongen and colleagues, now at Washington State University [14], was largely based on findings using the Psychomotor Vigilance Test (PVT), a reaction time test very sensitive to sleepiness (see Sect. 8.3 for a more detailed description) and subjective sleepiness using the SSS (see critique of SSS in Sect. 1.13). I will dwell on this study for a while, as it has had quite an impact on sleep research, being frequently used in supporting the sleep debt argument. Moreover, the findings can be interpreted from quite contrasting viewpoints, as will be seen.

A group of 48 healthy adult good sleepers, usually sleeping 7½–8 hours a night, were confined to the laboratory throughout the study, having been assigned to four equal groups, with their sleep restricted respectively to: 4, 6, or a control condition of 8 hours in bed, all maintained for 14 nights, with a fourth group totally sleep deprived for 3 nights (i.e. 88 hours continuous wakefulness). The actual total sleep times per night for the first three groups averaged 3.7, 5.5 and

6.6 hours respectively. For example the 8-hours-in-bed group were awake for 1.4 hours during this period. Participants underwent repeated PVTs and SSS measurements throughout the study. The 4- and 6-hour groups showed steady increases in subjective sleepiness over the first few days, which then levelled off. In contrast, the PVT scores (especially 'lapses') continued to worsen, with scores from the 4-hour group becoming greater than for the 6-hour group, as one might expect.

A critical finding was that by the end of the 14 days, the 6-hour group showed deteriorations in the PVT and SSS comparable to those who had been totally sleep deprived at the 2 night point, which led the investigators to conclude that "*since chronic sleep restriction to 6h per night produced cognitive performance deficits equivalent of up to two nights of total sleep deprivation, it appears that even moderate sleep restriction can seriously impair waking neurobehavioral functions in healthy adults ... Sleepiness ratings suggest that subjects were largely unaware of these increasing cognitive deficits, which may explain why the impact of chronic sleep restriction on waking cognitive functions is often assumed to be benign*" (p. 117).

Yet, one can argue that for the 6-hour sleep restricted group this effect was not equivalent to 2 nights of total sleep loss, as their sleep loss was actually double this amount and thus less debilitating than would be expected—for the following reason. As this group only obtained about 5.5 h sleep compared with their normally sleeping 8 hours per night, this gives a 2.4 hour nightly shortfall, which accumulates to 34 hours lost sleep over the 14 nights, whereas 2 nights without sleep for the zero-sleep group summates to about 15 hours of lost sleep; so these two conditions are not so equivalent, as more than double this sleep was lost during the 6-hour regimen. So, my alternative interpretation is that the 6-hour restricted group must have developed some adaptation to the sleep restriction, as despite their performance impairment being similar to that of 2 nights sleep deprivation, it should have been much worse, comparable to 4 nights without sleep.

Interestingly and unexpectedly, the 8-hour group also showed a small but steady increase in 'lapses' during the PVT, which led the investigators to conclude that this group also had insufficient sleep, and that their optimal sleep should have been 8.17 hours per night, in contrast with their home sleep logs before the study, showing an average sleep duration of 7.6 hours per night. Moreover, although they were in the study's 8-hour group, they had only been sleeping for 6.6 hours, an hour less than when at home.

In sum, this study advocated that we need around 8 hours' sleep, and that, in effect, sleep restricted to 6 hours (or rather 5.5 hours) is severely debilitating in terms of sleep loss. However, outside the laboratory, 8 hours' sleep seems to have been excess for these normally quite alert participants, and that 14 days of 5.5 hours' sleep was probably not so debilitating (albeit inadvisable) as claimed. Adaptation to shortened sleep is usually reflected by more intense SWS, and seen with increased 'Process S' at the beginning of sleep after sleep deprivation, seen in Fig. 6.2, earlier. I have rather laboured over this otherwise commendable study, because it is such a good example of how the same data can be interpreted in almost opposite ways, which happens in many areas of good science.

There have been several earlier, much longer, chronic sleep reduction studies, indicating that within limits we can adapt to less sleep, cf. [1], but these have not been well controlled, and I shall pass over them fairly quickly. Suffice to say that the best known and most substantial of these [15] required 8 healthy 7–8 hour sleeping young adults to reduce their daily sleep by 30 minutes every 2–4 weeks until they could go no further, which was about 5.5 hours, and confirmed by all-night sleep EEGs. The remarkable finding was not so much this part of the study, but that 8 months after it had ended, when the participants were free to sleep as they wished, they continued to average at least an hour less daily sleep than their original baseline levels, with their daytime alertness, efficiency at work, and all other aspects of behaviour being apparently quite normal. Their follow-up sleep EEGs showed their sleep to contain greater amounts of SWS and, in effect, they had lost their original last hour of sleep.

This apparent adaptation to long-term, reasonable reductions in sleep without harmful effects, is an example of 'allostasis', a well-known biological phenomenon whereby an organism can undergo physiological changes over time, and adapt to more efficient use. This is seen in the sleep of laboratory rodents. For example [16], when their usual daily sleep was curtailed for several days it became more intense in terms of

SWS. Subsequently, when allowed ad lib sleep, they showed little evidence of a sleep rebound to recover what was lost. To quote the authors: *"After losing approximately 35 h of sleep over 5 days of sleep restriction, animals regained virtually none of their lost sleep, even during a full 3-day recovery period"* (p. 10697).

6.6 Napping and Siestas

Thomas Edison was not only renowned for his numerous inventions, including the electric light, but for the numerous published pictures (for which he seemed to welcome) of him lying napping either in his famous office 'cots' or elsewhere in various unseemly places, such as on a workbench, under trees, even lying asleep on the lawn of US President Warren Harding's summer retreat, with the President sitting in a deckchair reading a newspaper and overlooking the somnolent Edison. Despite being so dismissive of sleep Edison was a prolific napper, always taking one or two short naps each day, lasting 20–30 minutes, then waking up quite refreshed, without grogginess and ready to go.

Yet, he was a fairly normal napper and, like the rest of us, by taking one or two of these short, timely naps we might well need only 5–6 hours' sleep at night. That is, by splitting daily sleep up this way, then the total amount of sleep needed per 24 hours will be reduced from that required during a single sleep of, say, 7 hours at night. This is why, in the population studies described earlier (Sects. 2.2 and 3.3), any failure to include possible daytime naps for those seemingly short 5-hour nighttime sleepers would have been an important oversight. However, the extent of this potentially beneficial effect of naps also depends on the duration of the nap as well as its regularity, as will be seen.

We can take more inspiration from Winston Churchill who declared that *"Nature has not intended mankind to work from eight in the morning until midnight without that refreshment of blessed oblivion which, even if it only lasts twenty minutes, is sufficient to renew all the vital forces."* Later, when he was asked by a journalist, *"To what do you attribute your success in life, sir"* Sir Winston replied, *"Conservation of energy. Never stand up when you can sit down. And never sit down when you can lie down."* A related, notable quote of his was "*You must sleep sometime between lunch and dinner, and no half-way measures. Take off your clothes and get into bed. That's what I always do. Don't think you will be doing less work because you sleep during the day. That's a foolish notion held by people who have no imagination. You will be able to accomplish more. You get two days in one—well, at least one and a half, I'm sure*", cf. [17].

However, in the UK few working people below retirement age have the opportunity to take a daytime nap other than occasionally at weekends and on days off. In hotter climates it is customary to have an afternoon siesta lasting for an hour or so, which for us is still reflected by that afternoon dip. That is, our circadian clock is ideally designed for two sleeps a day, a main sleep at night and a short one within the dip, and this is why, after a poor night's sleep, sleepiness and the likelihood of nodding off, is most likely then. This is more so in the elderly, as the mechanisms underlying the control of sleep and wakefulness also age, to the extent that their wakefulness cannot be sustained so easily for around 16 hours without a sleep, hence an afternoon nap, and maybe another nap early evening. Consequently they have a lesser need for sleep at night, maybe only 5 hours, depending on the duration of the naps. This, coupled with an early bedtime, leads to early morning awaking, and the inability to return to sleep as the need to sleep is complete. As I mentioned earlier (Sect. 1.9), this creates problems for the elderly when using sleeping tablets. Moreover, their afternoon naps are usually well beyond 20 minutes, to develop into more substantive sleep, and thus lessening nighttime sleep need.

This roughly 20-minute nap limit applies to us all, and can be very refreshing, without affecting nighttime sleep, whereas longer routine naps, as with a daily siesta, become part of the overall daily sleep requirement, and even reduce the duration of night sleep by longer than the siesta itself. For example, a regular one-hour siesta will shorten night sleep by about 90 minutes, as this is a more efficient way of distributing sleep over the day. In hot climates, the siesta also has the advantages of avoiding the heat of the early afternoon sun, and provides for more waking time in the cooler evenings.

In extreme cases people have adopted 'polyphasic sleep' by sleeping for around 60–90 minutes, usually four times a day, thus reducing daily sleep need to less than 6 hours rather than the usual, single 7 or so hours at night. Clearly this is not very practical, but is useful in emergencies, and can be continued for many weeks with little by way of heightened sleepiness during the waking periods. Long-distance lone sailors have utilised this method, described in an excellent book on the topic [18].

We [19] compared the effects of an early afternoon short nap with other methods for maintaining daytime alertness. A group of 20 carefully screened (by MSLTs and PVTs), young adult healthy good sleepers (average 7.6 hours sleep a night) who usually experienced only a modest afternoon dip, underwent four conditions a week apart, in random order:

1. 90 minutes extra time in bed in the morning, having been encouraged to carry on sleeping.
2. Usual night sleep plus a 20 minute afternoon nap at 2.30 p.m.
3. Usual night sleep plus 150 mg caffeine added to decaffeinated coffee given at 1.45 p.m.
4. A control condition of usual sleep plus this decaffeinated coffee (no extra caffeine).

Subjective sleepiness (the KSS), MSLTs and longer (20 minute) reaction time tests (PVTs—see Sect. 8.3) were measured from 4 p.m. every two hours until 10 p.m.

The morning sleep group increased this sleep by an average of 74 minutes, and all the nap group were able to nap for 15–20 minutes. Compared with the control condition, all three of the active treatments (1-3 above) reduced afternoon and evening sleepiness, seen in all the measures, but with the nap being most effective, closely followed by the caffeine, and then the morning sleep extension. Again it could be argued that our participants might have previously experienced some 'sleep debt', given they were able to extend morning sleep, but this was the poorest of the treatments, in only nominally improving their overall MSLT scores (averaging 1.5 minutes). Interestingly, the caffeine was almost as good as the nap. But it was clear that this timely short nap was indeed better than the more lengthy extended sleep. Moreover, given the relatively poor effect of the extended sleep, this again indicates that this extra sleep was largely beyond any real sleep need.

Let me now end this topic of napping with some further aspects of interest.

Until recently, daytime napping was often seen as some sort of 'weakness', and more as a characteristic of the elderly. But thanks to naps now being rebranded as 'powernaps', despite being exactly the same as the traditional nap, napping is back in vogue, with greater appeal especially with young men who can even brag about its virtues.

A rapid, tried and tested [20] 30-minute method for overcoming moderate sleepiness is to combine the caffeine with a nap, but not in the usual way. First, have about 150 mg of caffeine, for example, as usually found with two rounded 5 ml teaspoons of coffee granules. Because caffeine usually takes around 20 minutes to have effect, here is the ideal window of opportunity for that short 15–20 minute nap, taken immediately after the coffee. Then allow a few minutes to 'freshen up'. Their combined actions can be very effective for some hours.

Finally, I must emphasise that the irregular, occasional nap has to be kept short, ideally less than 20 minutes, otherwise it develops into a full-blown sleep, leading to that post sleep inertia. Naps can be much longer, without subsequent grogginess, if taken at the same time, every day, as in a regular siesta and thus integrated into one's total daily sleep requirement.

6.7 Summing Up

All biological needs are flexible, within limits, able to be reduced or taken to excess, as in eating without hunger (with a 'hearty appetite'), and in drinking for pleasure, without thirst. Similarly, we can sleep in excess of its need, for enjoyment, reflecting an 'appetite for sleep' rather than a 'sleep hunger'. Thus 'sleeping to excess' is not necessarily synonymous with recovery from sleep debt, as there may well be little or nothing to repay, as 'sleep debt' usually denies the ability to sleep from boredom or just for pleasure. On the other hand, as was seen with those seasonal changes to sleep (described in Sect. 2.3), and when pressures for wakefulness are greater, we have the ability to adapt to somewhat shorter sleep, given the time in which to do it, and without apparently increasing daytime sleepiness.

The functions of sleep that are most essential to survival will be particularly evident at its beginning, presumably reflected by SWS (and Process S), tailing off as sleep progresses, to a point where the rise in our circadian clock acts as sleep's terminator. Nevertheless, the latter can be 'consciously' overridden and, within limits, we can continue to sleep 'at leisure', depending on the various impositions of one's wakefulness. Chapter 13 describes how REM towards the end of the night has this capacity for flexibility, being a 'buffer' between wakefulness and non-REM sleep.

That sleep quality is probably as important as its quantity, is also seen in recovery sleep after total sleep loss, when less than half of the lost sleep needs to be reclaimed, mainly as SWS. Moreover, sleeping just once a day, in a single uninterrupted block at night, as is our custom, usually requires more total daily sleep than when distributing sleep somewhat over the 24 hours. It will be remembered (Sect. 1.12) that it was once common to split nighttime sleep into 'first' and 'second' sleeps. Short naps and longer siestas can be most cost-effective time-wise, albeit for somewhat different reasons, but represent what might well be the more natural and efficient way for distributing our daily sleep. All of which again suggest that sleep debt in terms of the duration of a night's sleep, as well as the concept of 'social jet lag', may not be so problematic as is often assumed.

6.8   Sleepless in New Jersey

So, to end on another, lighter historical note. Everyone sleeps and needs to do so but, nevertheless, and over the last hundred years or so newspapers have latched on to claims from various individuals that they have not slept for years, and seem none the worse for it. In February 1904 *The New York Times* published a special report on Albert E Herpin, a stableman, who *"hasn't slept a wink during the last ten years"* and that this had been corroborated by physicians. *"He is in perfect health and does not seem to suffer any discomfort ... goes to bed regularly but says he never closes his eyes* or at least never for an instant loses consciousness of all going on around him. In the morning he rises refreshed and ready for another day's work among the horses. He declares the change of position and the darkness of the room seem to give him all the rest he requires." Apparently it all began when his son was born, and "kept him walking the floor at nights" and, according to physicians who examined him, "his nervous system was shattered by this experience". Sadly, his wife died shortly afterwards and he became a widower. Several further accounts followed and by August "he refuses offers from all parts of the world to exhibit himself", including "$10,000 from a Viennese scientific association to undergo a 30 days' test of his ability to live without sleep". This was a huge sum of course, and the reason papers didn't become even more suspicious must fall under that rather maligned press rubric of 'never let the truth get in the way of a good story'.

His notoriety quickly spread, and apparently not only did he receive a letter from President Teddy Roosevelt inviting him to come to Washington, as the President wanted to "shake the hand of a wide awake republican", but he had 14 leap-year proposals of marriage. In fact, a wealthy widow from New York, after writing two letters to the "sleepless wonder", and getting no reply, came to find him, and after personally proposing marriage went back home disappointed. Apparently he had declared that reporters, museum managers and doctors were bad enough to contend with, but that "these leap-year propositions are the limit". As one might expect, he also received many letters from jokers giving advice on how to sleep, including, "before retiring, blow out the gas" (lighting was by coal gas), and "reverse yourself in bed, let your head hang over the footboard and place your feet on the pillow" as it was thought by many at the time that increasing blood to the head induced sleep.

He died in 1947 aged over 90, apparently of heart failure and seemingly still sleepless all these years, but never having had his claims independently verified to anyone's satisfaction. Nevertheless, according to The New York Times of 24 February that year, he was still respected as a "local scientific wonder … always getting his rest while wide awake sitting upright in a chair".

Other entertaining accounts, at the time, of other seemingly sleepless people from outside the USA, could be found in the world's press, which also attracted much attention especially in the USA. For example, in 1938 the *Milwaukee Chronicle* reported on the "Sleepless Man—Still a Puzzle", Paul Kern, a Hungarian soldier, who, in 1915 during the First World War, had apparently been shot through the temple. He seemed to recover quite quickly, but could no longer sleep, and thus attracted much press coverage in Hungary and elsewhere, as a cause célèbre, having been dubbed the "*citizen who never sleeps*", and who apparently remained sleepless right up to his death in 1955. After having recovered from his war wound, he worked for the Hungarian government, maintaining good health, apart from "the occasional headache". His X-rays had not shown much, if anything, of brain damage, which is surprising, although X-ray methods were not as sophisticated as they are today. Sleeping pills apparently had no effect, neither did alcohol, which he "*only tried twice, and made him more wakeful than ever*". At nights he maintained a fixed routine whereby he went to cafés (we have no idea what he drank there), walked and read books until 2 a.m. and, on the advice of his doctors sat and relaxed for one hour, keeping his eyes closed but "*hopelessly could not sleep*", supposedly demonstrated by his smoking a pipe which, according to various observers, "*continued to glow*" throughout this eyes-closed period. At 3 a.m. he was off walking again, usually in parks to talk to his "*beggared friends, who sleep there … and to the poor huddled in doorways*". He would have eight meals per 24 hours, not counting snacks. Despite the attention of numerous specialist clinicians, including hypnotists, all of whom tried to cure Kern of his 'mysterious disease', all failed.

References

1. Horne JA. 1988 *Why We Sleep*. Oxford: University Press.
2. Lamond N et al 2008 The dynamics of neurobehavioural recovery following sleep loss. *J Sleep Res*, 16, 33–41.
3. Borbely AA 1982 A two process model of sleep regulation. *Human Neurobiology*, 1, 195–204.
4. Aserinsky E. 1969 The maximal capacity for sleep: Rapid eye movement density as an index of sleep satiety. *Biol Psychiat*. 1: 147–159.
5. Aserinsky E. 1973 Relationship of rapid eye movement density to the prior accumulation of sleep and wakefulness. *Psychophysiol*. 10: 545–558.

6. Roehrs T et al 1989 Sleep extension in sleepy and alert normals. *Sleep.* 12: 449–457.

7. Harrison Y, Horne JA. 1996 Long-term extension to sleep - are we chronically sleep deprived? *Psychophysiol.* 33: 22–30.

8. Horne JA. 2010 Sleepiness as a need for sleep: when is enough, enough? Neurosci Biobehav Rev 34: 108–118.

9. Rattenborg NC et al 2008 Sleeping outside the box: electroencephalographic measures of sleep in sloths inhabiting a rainforest. *Biol Lett.* 4: 402–405.

10. Palmer CD et al 1980 Sleep patterns and life style in Oxfordshire villages. *J Biosoc Sci*, 12: 437–467.

11. National Sleep Foundation SF (2003) http://www.sleepfoundation.org/polls/2003SleepPollExecSumm.pdf.

12. Wittmann M et al. 2006 Social jetlag: misalignment of biological and social time *Chronobiol Int.* 23:497–509.

13. Roenneberg T et al 2012 Social jetlag and obesity *Curr Biol.* 22:939–943.

14. Van Dongen HP et al 2003 The cumulative cost of additional wakefulness: Dose-response effects on neurobehavioral functions and sleep physiology from chronic sleep restriction and total sleep deprivation. *Sleep.* 26: 117–126.

15. Mullaney DJ et al 1977. Sleep during and after gradual sleep reduction. Psychophysiol, 14: 237–244.

16. Kim Y et al 2007. Repeated sleep restriction in rats leads to homeostatic and allostatic responses during recovery sleep. *Proc Natl Acad Sci U S A.* 104:10697–10702.

17. Graebner W 1965 *My Dear Mister Churchill*, Boston: Houghton Mifflin Co.

18. Stampi C 1992. *Why We Nap*. Boston-Birkhäuser.

19. Horne JA et al 2008 Sleep extension versus nap or coffee, within the context of sleep extension. J Sleep Res 17: 432–436.

20. Reyner LA & Horne JA 1997 Suppression of sleepiness in drivers: combination of caffeine with a short nap. *Psychophysiology*, 34: 721–725.

7

Illumination

7.1 Enlightenment

Of all the inputs into the human brain, from all the senses, one-third comes from our eyes, which is proportionately much greater than for the eyes of most other mammals. Moreover, our visual system is particularly highly developed, especially for seeing colour, and heavily reliant on daylight until the advent of artificial lighting (e.g. oil-lamps) which only appeared very recently in our evolution. Daylight and even regular exposure to artificial light (especially if it has a blue tinge) are critical time setters for our circadian clock, although in the absence of these light sources, we have other albeit less powerful external 'time-givers' (otherwise known as 'zeitgebers'), including regular daily events such as mealtimes, the morning alarm clock and daily set social events.

This particular light perception comes from recently discovered 'non-seeing' cells in the retina, quite distinct from the rods and cones integral to our sense of sight, and most sensitive to blue light. They detect light 'unconsciously' and signal its presence to the suprachiasmatic nucleus (SCN) within the brain, it being the seat of the circadian pacemaker which in turn controls the nearby pineal gland and its release of the

© The Editor(s) (if applicable) and The Author(s) 2016
J. Horne, *Sleeplessness*, DOI 10.1007/978-3-319-30572-1_7

hormone melatonin into the bloodstream for distribution throughout the body. All body cells have individual circadian clocks that are synchronised largely at the behest of melatonin, the 'circadian messenger'. Melatonin is the 'hormone of the night', and is suppressed by daylight as well as by bright artificial light. As it is produced by all mammals during the night, even for those that are nocturnally active, melatonin is not really a sleep inducer as is often thought, but indicates when to sleep and when to wake rather than how to sleep.

Bright indoor light at night also has a separate, more rapid alerting action on other parts of the brain, unrelated to the circadian clock, independent of melatonin suppression, and effective for night workers trying to remain awake. Daylight and bright indoor light also reduce daytime sleepiness and the propensity to nap in the daytime. This is particularly helpful in those elderly people prone to sleeping too much in the day with consequently poorer sleep at night, as this light helps shorten the naps, to concentrate night sleep. This method is also effective with babies, as by letting them have their daytime naps in the light, not in a darkened room, also shortens these naps and so lengthens their night sleep, usually with fewer awakenings. However, this method is not effective until about 3–4 months of age, by which time their circadian clock has become more apparent.

In Sect. 2.3 I described the relatively little impact of seasonal changes in daylight on sleep on today's industrial societies even for those above the Arctic Circle, where there is over 20 hours difference in daily daylight between summer and winter, but more than adequate artificial lighting. Nevertheless, sleep was one hour longer in the winter [1]. On the other hand, for those more 'natural' non-industrial societies without artificial light, living near the equator, where the seasonal differences in daylight are fairly small, the one-hour seasonal difference in sleep duration seems comparable with a similar change in daylight. However, even here there are other accompanying influences on sleep and wakefulness, especially with changing food availability, environmental temperature and other weather effects. Consequently, under these natural settings it is difficult to ascribe seasonal effects on sleep solely to changes in daylight.

7.2   Curtains

In the UK, with its roughly 8-hour seasonal difference in daylight, and maybe thanks to dark curtains in the summer mornings and evenings, and artificial light in the winter, as well as to other constraints on our time, such as work, school and commuting times, there is little by way of any seasonal change to today's westernised sleep. Of course, a sudden shift in daylight and one-hour loss of sleep, as can happen when the clocks go forward with daylight saving time (DST) in the spring, also require adjustment of sleep, with some temporary consequences [2]. In the UK [3] more road accidents occur in these initial few days, arguably due to shorter sleep, and in the USA [4], on the Mondays following this switch to DST, there are more workplace injuries, whereas on the Mondays after the switch to winter time, with a one-hour gain, there are no such effects.

Worry that DST might lead to more accidents goes back well over a hundred years, and was one of many arguments used against its initiation. In the UK it was first proposed by the enthusiastic William Willett to "*improve health and happiness*". He was a wealthy builder who, in 1907, and at his own expense, produced the pamphlet, "Waste of Daylight", distributed widely, including to politicians, town councils and businesses. In it he wrote, "*That so many as 210 hours of daylight are to all intents and purposes wasted every year, is a defect in our civilisation. Let England recognise and remedy it. Let us not be so faint-hearted as to hesitate to make the effort when the cost is too trifling and the reward so great*". Inspiring stuff, and just a sample of what he wrote.

Mindful of sudden changes, he suggested adding 20 minutes to clocks each Sunday night for four consecutive weeks in the spring, accumulating to 80 minutes of daylight saving per day, and then to reverse this in the autumn. He even provided a detailed cost-benefit analysis, calculating that DST would save precisely £2,546,834 annually for the whole nation. Nevertheless, it was ridiculed at first, despite the support of the young politician at the time, Winston Churchill, and the influential author Sir Arthur Conan Doyle. Unfortunately Willett never lived to see DST becoming law, as he died of influenza in 1915. Ironically, the next year DST was introduced as an emergency wartime measure, throughout Europe (even in Germany where it had been introduced on orders of Kaiser Wilhelm II), but was then dropped after the war, only to be gradually reintroduced. Sadly, Willett's efforts are mostly forgotten, except in his home town of Pitts Wood, Kent, where there is a memorial sundial set permanently to DST and a pub, *The Daylight Inn*.

In 1968 the UK changed to continuous summer time throughout the year, mainly for commercial reasons. But due to public pressure, mostly from those living in the north, the government abandoned it in 1972, reverting back to DST, with British Summer Time (BST) in the summer and Greenwich Mean Time (GMT) for the winter.

7.3   Larks and Owls

Our circadian clock is not the same for everyone and there are natural variations in the timing of the daily peaks and troughs, to the extent that we can be loosely divided up into 'chronotypes' [5]. Put more simply, some of us are 'larks' or 'morning types' feeling at one's daily best in the mornings, whereas 'owls' or 'evening types' are at their best in the evenings. In wanting to get up later in the morning the owl has a poor appetite then, whereas the lark can enjoy a 'hearty breakfast'. Around 20 % of adults are what I describe as either definite owls or larks, about 40 % are neither one nor the other, and the remaining 40 % are either moderate larks or moderate owls [5]. Figure 7.1 shows these approximate circadian differences in alertness in 20–30 year old definite morning and evening types.

Irrespective of being a lark or owl, we are at our most 'owlish' in the late teens, to become more 'larkish' as we get older. Although the lark is also an earlier riser than the owl, who stays up and goes to bed later, their sleep lengths are about the same. However, the circadian early morning body temperature trough is about two hours later for the owl. Interestingly, there is a hereditary aspect to being an owl or lark, with at least one gene being identified, known as 'Period-3' ('Per-3'), having 'long' and 'short' variants with the former tending to identify larks and the latter owls.

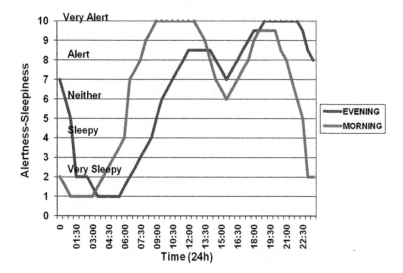

Fig. 7.1 Typical circadian differences in alertness for 'definite' morning and evening types

Some years ago we designed a simple 19-item questionnaire [5], still in frequent use throughout the world, and translated into many languages. Owls are generally better able than larks at adapting to changes in the timing of their sleep, as happens with DST, shift work and jet lag. They tend to be the more extrovert creative types, more sociable and people-oriented. Seemingly, they are more likely to be the poets, artists and inventors, while the larks tend to be rather more conformist, punctual and think more logically. There are many sayings relating to owls and larks. Ambrose Bierce in his *Devil's Dictionary* believed that *"dawn is when men of reason go to bed"*, and although Dr Samuel Johnson noted *"whoever goes to bed before midnight is a rogue"*, he is also attributed to saying *"nobody who does not rise early will ever do any good"*, which was rather hypocritical as he would often stay in bed until midday.

We hear that *"the early bird catches the worm"* (unattributed) and that in 1735 the American polymath Benjamin Franklin noted in *Poor Richard's Almanack* that, *"early to bed and early to rise, makes a man healthy wealthy and wise*". Various studies have put this often irritating viewpoint to the test, and failed to support it. Probably the most intriguing study was that published in the British Medical Journal [6]. Here, 1299 men and women aged 65 and over had taken part in a UK Department of Health survey on many aspects of health, including sleeping patterns, socio-economic circumstances including income and type of accommodation, as well as cognitive function. Of these, 29 % were defined as larks (bed before 11 p.m. and up before 8 a.m.) and 26 % as owls (both bed and getting up times being later), with the remaining 45 % being neither type. There was no evidence to show that larks were any more affluent, in fact it was the owls who had the larger ongoing income and better cars. Neither were there differences in their self-reported sleeping patterns, nor sleep durations and cognitive abilities. Both types had a slightly lower risk of death 23 years later, which was attributed to their spending less time in bed compared with neither types. Despite there being only one of the cognitive measures alluding to 'wisdom', it did not differ between the two types. Maybe, though, other sleep-related proverbs might make much better sense, such as, "*not burning the candle at both ends*".

7.4   Jet Lag

This temporary misalignment of the usual timing of sleep due to a shift in local time takes longer to adjust when travelling eastwards, owing to a shortened day, whereas with westbound travel it is easier for the circadian clock to adapt to the lengthened day. However, there are complications depending on whether flights are overnight, causing poor sleep and a desire to go to bed soon after arrival, as can happen when flying from the USA to the UK. In which case, and ideally, one should have no more than an hour's sleep that morning, then use caffeine and daylight until the evening. Although sleep might come easily that first night, the next morning's wakening (e.g. 7 a.m.) will be difficult, being around midnight in the USA. By getting up and utilising caffeine (as in coffee) and daylight once more, both will promote alertness. Melatonin as a tablet (e.g. 3 mg) taken soon after sunset may help to advance the otherwise delayed sleep into the earlier evening, providing that bright light is avoided, but the

7 a.m. subsequent wake-up has to be maintained. This regimen following west to east travel, of evening melatonin, with a stable morning wake-up time followed by plenty of light will help accelerate the re-establishment of both the body clock and sleep within local time.

Flights from the UK to the USA mostly depart around midday, arriving about mid-afternoon local time, which is evening in the UK. In this situation, sleep should be avoided until local evening and, instead, use daylight ideally with some caffeine until then, when sleepiness will likely demand bedtime and sleep by around 9 p.m. local time. The subsequent waking up in the small hours of the local time (morning in the UK) is not easily rectified by a sleeping tablet taken then, as a high dose is usually needed, liable to cause grogginess later that morning. A better solution, given that it is still dark at this early hour in the USA, is to avoid bright indoor light and take a melatonin tablet (e.g. 3 mg) as this will help trick the circadian clock into extending its night. During the following day (US local time), one or two short (15 minute) naps will help, together with caffeine and daylight, helping one to keep awake well into the evening with the aid of bright indoor lighting. A melatonin tablet should be avoided until awakening in the early hours, as before. To recap on taking melatonin: westbound travel, take it on unwanted early (local) morning awakening; eastbound travel, take it early (local) evening, just after sunset. It is very important to obtain melatonin tablets from a reputable source.

7.5   Shift Work

About 17 % of working adults in the western world work shifts, including nights. Moreover, many people increasingly work from home in the evenings and weekends, when work and rest can often merge. Nevertheless, most shifts, whether they be 8, 10 or, increasingly nowadays, 12 hours long, usually change every 2–3 days, causing disruptions of sleep and to the circadian rhythm, as well as with family and social life. Such effects combine into a mixture of 'sleepiness', 'tiredness' and 'fatigue' as I described in Chap. 1, often causing additional stress, and hence the need for adequate rest days, away from work. Following three successive 12-hour night shifts, comprising 'compressed weeks', the associated rest days can entail four days off, which can be quite tempting. However, as up to two of these days are needed for recovery, then at least one of them ought to be considered as a 'work but without work' day. On the other hand, these rest days can just provide for 'moonlighting' at other jobs.

Long work hours are not intrinsically harmful if there is good job satisfaction, and in these respects there is no difference between 8- and 12-hour shifts [7], usually indicated by low absenteeism. Besides, adequate company occupational health services, family support, good coping strategies, an attractive work environment, friendly colleagues, supportive bosses, sufficient rest breaks, plenty of work variety with low monotony, an ability to plan one's work schedule (even with a demanding job), all contribute to maintaining good mental and physical health during many years of shift working.

Although there are findings of higher incidences of cardiovascular disease, hypertension and obesity related disorders amongst shift workers, it usually take several years of working in this way before any symptoms may develop. Thus, one cannot attribute such adverse effects to shift work alone and, more to the point, to disrupted sleep, as there are those other various aspects, and the extent to which the work itself is stressful versus satisfying. Other, more indirect and undesirable effects of this lifestyle include a poor diet (e.g. too much junk food), too little exercise and a greater likelihood of smoking and consuming alcohol. Moreover, there are individual differences in coping, including being an owl, who seems better able to adapt and cope than the lark. Age is another factor, as not only are younger adults more owl-like and thus more adaptable, but older shift workers tend to have greater problems with sleeping by day. On the other hand, older workers may have the experience of developing better coping strategies for dealing with their shift work.

Many companies adopt 'Fatigue Risk Management Systems' [7] for employees, utilising various tried and tested occupational health techniques, including well-designed shift-rostering methods, helping to minimise adverse effects of shift work on worker well-being. These are usually very cost-effective in having the benefits of improving productivity and reducing absenteeism.

In terms of sleepiness and sleep, helpful advice for night-shift workers includes working under reasonably bright light (ideally blue tinged), sufficient to suppress melatonin levels and to increase alertness, as well as utilising short (15 minute) naps during rest breaks. Better still, utilise that coffee (caffeine) immediately followed by a nap method, described earlier (Sect. 6.6). Further advice is to delay going straight to bed immediately on arriving back home in the morning if there is another night shift to follow, as this sleep will be short and unsatisfactory due to the morning rise in the circadian clock promoting wakefulness (as in the 'two process model', 6.2). Although many people will resort to sleeping tablets in attempting to counteract this poorer daytime sleep, higher doses are required with the risk of excessive subsequent grogginess. A better, longer sleep will be gained if it is delayed until after midday (maybe caffeine and light to keep awake until then), to coincide with the afternoon dip, which also avoids using sleeping tablets. An added benefit is that the nearer this sleep is to the next night shift, the less will be sleepiness that night. Finally, morning shifts ought not to be rostered to begin before 7.00 a.m., as this usually leads to excessive daytime sleepiness [10] owing to too early a morning rising, which is usually not compensated by an earlier bedtime the night before.

References

1. Kleitman N, Kleitman H. 1953.The sleep-wakefulness pattern in the Arctic. *Scientific Monthly*, 76, 349–356.
2. Harrison Y 2013 The impact of daylight saving time on sleep and related behaviours. *Sleep Med Rev* 17: 285–292.
3. Monk TH, Folkard S. 1976 Adjusting to the changes to and from Daylight Saving Time. *Nature*. 261:688–689.
4. Barnes CM, Wagner DT 2009 Changing to daylight saving time cuts into sleep and increases workplace injuries. *J Appl Psychol* 94: 1305–1317.
5. Horne JA, Ostberg O. 1976 A self-assessment questionnaire to determine morningness-eveningness in human circadian rhythms *Int J Chronobiol*. 4:97–110.
6. Gale C, Martyn C 1998. Larks and owls and health, wealth, and wisdom *Br Med J* 317:1675–7.
7. Tucker P, Folkard S 2012. ILO *Working Time, Health and Safety – a Research Synthesis Paper*. ILO, Geneva.

8

Sleepiness

8.1 Implications

A sleepiness, unnoticeable in the everyday life of healthy good sleepers can easily appear during the daytime when we comfortably sit for, say, half an hour under dull and boring circumstances, quite safe and with no pressure to do anything else, when it is quite possible that we would then allow ourselves to fall asleep. However, new and interesting stimulation will rapidly alleviate this sleepiness, as can standing up and walking off. Is such a sleepiness, unnoticeable in everyday activities, eked out by boredom, just created *de novo* by this boredom or a sign of hidden 'sleep debt'? Whereas in some cases the latter will be true, sleepiness may not necessarily be indicative of sleep loss, but an 'appetitive sleepiness', comparable to having an appetite for food when satiated and without a feeling of hunger, but stimulated by the sight of attractive food. On the other hand, we can simply decide to ignore this temptation and forget it. More about appetitive sleepiness and its consequential 'sleepability', in a moment.

Sleep research devotes much effort into the topic of sleepiness and its measurement, especially as it is so integral to the sleep debt debate, and

© The Editor(s) (if applicable) and The Author(s) 2016
J. Horne, *Sleeplessness*, DOI 10.1007/978-3-319-30572-1_8

associated claims that people may not realise how sleepy they might be [1, 2]. Although sleepiness is indeed an important aspect of sleep, the impression might be given that the primary role of sleep is mostly to eliminate sleepiness. A parallel can be drawn with eating, which is not just for overcoming hunger, as the different constituents of food, such as carbohydrates, proteins, fat and so on, play subtle and vital roles, as probably do the different EEG constituents of sleep. Whereas sleepiness, of whatever sort, can be suppressed to some extent, at least temporarily, by a relatively simple substance such as caffeine, this contrasts with the large number of complex substances and mechanisms in the brain that produce and regulate sleep itself, which again suggests that sleepiness, at least in its more noticeable form, is only one of a variety of symptoms of any sleep loss, albeit the most obvious and fairly easy to measure—maybe all too easy. As will be seen, sleepiness can be detected to varying extents by different measures, depending on: the type of test, its duration, the dullness of the environment, the extent to which participants can go at their own pace, their belief in the purpose of the test, whether they are compliant or otherwise decide to put effort into counteracting any sleepiness, and any external incentives.

8.2   Falling Asleep Versus Staying Awake

The Multiple Sleep Latency Test (MSLT) was briefly described earlier (Sect. 1.6) and is a most useful test of sleepiness, used under clinical and experimental settings. To recap on the test [3], participants attend a sleep centre, and at two hourly intervals, usually from 10 a.m. to 4 p.m. or maybe 6 p.m., they lie down on a comfortable bed in a quiet and darkened room and are asked to 'relax and try and go to sleep'. Their EEGs are monitored and the first sign of sleep lasting beyond 15 seconds is taken as sleep onset, and the session is terminated. Or, if by 20 minutes if there is no sign of sleep then sleep onset is usually assumed to be 20 minutes. The average sleep onset time for these sessions gives the MSLT score, with scores lower than 10–12 minutes seen to be indicative of some level of 'excessive' sleepiness. At least half of normal adults, without sleep complaints, having had their usual amount of sleep, will fall asleep (according to the 15 second criterion) within the 20-minute limit of a MSLT session, although, of course, this likelihood is higher during early afternoon sessions.

If these sessions are extended to 30 minutes, then most people will indeed fall asleep, which shows just how many of us can fairly easily fall asleep during the daytime, given the right circumstances. But whether this is still illustrative of hidden 'sleep debt' is another matter. One of the best examples comes from a large study [4] of 100 volunteers, equal numbers of men and women, aged 25–65 years. All were screened to exclude sleep complaints and any subjective signs of even minor daytime sleepiness, and who had maintained their usual sleep habits for two weeks prior to undergoing a day of five MSLTs. However, these sessions were extended to 30 minutes, and of the total of 500 sessions, sleep onset occurred on 413 (83 %) occasions, and only two participants never fell asleep. The average MSLT scores were rather longer, as one might expect.

Nevertheless, one might ask why so many people can fall asleep at times of the day when they would not normally do so, and whether this indicates sleep debt having reached epidemic proportions. Or, on the other hand, maybe there is a voluntary ability to fall asleep under low levels of sleepiness, given the conducive circumstances to do so. One might call this 'high sleepability', which is distinct from needing sleep due to obviously insufficient sleep. When healthy participants, free of sleep disorders, come to a sleep laboratory they might have an expectancy to be somewhat sleepy, which can be likened to someone well satiated, neither hungry nor looking for food, then taken to an attractive café and confronted with aromas of fresh bread, croissants and so on, and presented with a choice of these items. The likelihood is that an enticing item will be selected and soon eaten with relish. Was there an unmasked, hidden hunger after all, or was it just eating for pleasure [4]? Besides, we can eat simply out of boredom. Here, I see high sleepability and the decision actually to go to sleep as a 'conscious and voluntary' act following appetitive sleepiness.

Thus, a normal, healthy sleeper in a sleep laboratory, who is relaxed, maybe rather bored, with few interesting distractions and no waking pressures, will probably show that their most likely behaviour is a propensity to fall asleep, albeit after longer than the 12-minute criterion of 'excessive daytime sleepiness' but, nevertheless, even within 20 minutes. My point is that as sleepiness presumably appeared before this sleep onset, then it was likely to have been generated by the circumstances and one's volition rather than be indicative of any real need for sleep.

Not only is the MSLT very sensitive to sleepiness, even to very low levels that maybe only exist under exacting laboratory conditions, but the same can apply to the monotonous reaction time tests I will come to. Such levels of sleepiness can go unnoticed by and be of little concern to people during their everyday situations, who are not prepared to change their waking habits for more daily sleep, which would only provide minimal benefits in terms of greater waking alertness and productivity. Hence, it could be argued that people do not really know how sleepy they are, whereas these objective tests will indicate this.

There is a variant of the MSLT, the 'Maintenance of Wakeful Test' (MWT [3]), which is more real-world, where the participant sits in a reclining chair, wired up with an EEG, as with the MSLT, but in a quiet room, under brighter lighting, and this time is asked to 'try and stay awake'. The time taken to fall asleep is again measured, with the test ending if and when the participant falls asleep. Up to 40 minutes is allowed for each session, and like the MSLT, this test is also repeated four to five times every two hours from 10 a.m. The average time to fall asleep, in minutes, is the overall MWT score. Nil sleep is scored as 40 minutes. As might be expected, MWT scores are two to three times longer than those for the MSLT.

Despite these latter scores being longer, one might expect there to be a high correlation between the outcomes of the MSLT and MWT; that is, people who have low scores on one will have relatively low scores on the other, but this is not the case as the association is weak [4]. These two tests seemingly measure two semi-independent abilities—falling asleep and staying awake [5, 6].

One extreme example of this difference concerns those patients with obstructive sleep apnoea syndrome, causing them to have excessive daytime sleepiness (EDS, see Sect. 9.2), and unwanted (involuntary) episodes of falling asleep in the daytime. When successfully treated their nighttime sleep usually returns to normal, with no complaint or signs of daytime EDS. Nevertheless, they seem to be very sleepy when returning to the sleep clinic for a check-up, as their MSLT scores can remain very low [6, 7], as they fall asleep quickly when instructed to 'relax and try and go to sleep', as required by this test. But there is no other evidence of sleepiness and their MWT scores are usually normal [7]. So it seems that their many years of suffering from the disorder has left them with the ability to fall asleep rapidly if they so wish, but with little real sleepiness. Here, it seems that the process of instigating sleep is somewhat separate from sleepiness itself. For them, falling asleep can be a pre-meditated voluntary decision under much conscious control, presumably enabling them easily to fall asleep when asked to do so during the MSLT. That is, they seem to have 'high sleepability', in easily being able to fall asleep seemingly with minimal sleepiness if they so wish, whereas they are quite able to remain awake under 'awake-promoting' circumstances. Of course, at bedtime there is the usual sleepiness, which itself also promotes sleep. On the other hand, it seems that for many of those other people with insomnia, they are at the other extreme, in having 'poor sleepability', with their apparent inability to fall asleep.

8.3 Monotony

Arguably the other most commonly used test of sleepiness is the Psychomotor Vigilance Test (PVT) [1, 8]. It is a reaction time test whereby participants sit facing a computer screen, in a sound-dampened, small cubicle, with minimal visual distractions. The index finger of one's dominant hand rests on a button, ready to depress it in response to a digital millisecond clock that appears on the screen in random intervals of between 5 and 12 seconds. The response stops the clock, which remains in view for 1–2 seconds, to give the participant some feedback on their performance. Typically, the task lasts 10 minutes. Two main scores are usually obtained: the average reaction time of all responses less than 500 milliseconds, and the number of responses greater than 500 milliseconds, called 'lapses'. The longer the reaction time and the more the lapses, the greater is the sleepiness.

The PVT is particularly sensitive to 'lapses', that can last up to a few seconds, which not only consist of 'microsleeps', but also distractions from the screen, despite there being little around by way of distraction. Microsleeps are those gradually droopy eyelids and loss of responsiveness, typically followed by a shake of the head and a return to alertness for a minute or so until the process repeats itself. This drifting in and out of wakefulness is also what naturally happens when we close our eyes at bedtime to go to sleep, or rather 'drift in and out of sleep', when micro-sleeps rapidly become longer and longer, eventually coalescing to become sustained sleep.

Under these mundane testing conditions, when people are bored or sleepy and try to stay awake, the brain and behaviour need and seek stimulation. In looking away from the computer screen people can miss a signal which is recorded as a lapse. Under PVT scoring conditions maybe this does not really matter, as a distraction is probably as good as a micro-sleep in terms of a lapse. However, we [9, 10] found that this 'distractabil-ity' is itself an important measure, as it can reveal three different aspects of behaviour, as a result of: (1) otherwise alert boredom, merely looking away from the screen and missing a signal; (2) an actual microsleep; or (3) distraction due to more severe sleep loss, including attempts to seek some stimulation as a means of trying to stay awake; this latter aspect is covered in Sect. 11.2. All this points to the advisability of recording the participant's EEG as well as view their face via a camera, which together can distinguish between these three aspects. Simply measuring reaction times alone can miss these other important clues as to what is really going on.

Interestingly, reaction times do not generally slow down much with sleepiness, as is usually thought, as between lapses individual reactions are near normal, typically slowing by less than 100 milliseconds, whereas there is no reaction during a lapse, of course. However, if all the responses are averaged together, including those within lapses that might only occur every couple of minutes or so, and compared with a dozen normal responses, then the overall reaction time will appear significantly slower.

Although the MSLT and PVT are deemed to be objective tests of sleepiness, again, findings between them do not always concur, espe-cially as the PVT is 'experimenter-paced', unlike the 'subject-paced' MSLT. That is, the sudden appearance of a stimulus on a screen within the PVT setting is computer-generated and unpredictable (within limits), with the participant having no control over this. In contrast, if and when the participant falls asleep during the MSLT, this is at their own pace. Generally, experimenter-paced tasks are more sensitive to sleepiness than are subject-paced ones. Other influential differences between the PVT and MSLT are that the PVT involves sitting in a well-lit, small room with the participant encouraged to do their best at responding to the stimuli when these appear, whereas the MSLT entails the participant lying on a comfortable bed in a darkened room and encouraged to go to sleep. Thus, it is not surprising that these two tests produce different outcomes.

8.4   Subjective Sleepiness

Of the various sleepiness scales given to participants to rate their own sleepiness, the most coherent and unambiguous is the 9-point Karolinska Sleepiness Scale (KSS) [11], seen below. Earlier (Sect. 1.13), I described the often used Stanford Sleepiness Scale (SSS) that contains too many ambiguities. There are also alternative 'analogue' sleepiness scales, having a 10 cm line 'anchored' at either end by the terms 'very alert' or 'very sleepy', requiring a cross to be placed at an appropriate point along the scale, with the distance in millimetres along the scale indicating the level of perceived sleepiness.

Karolinska Sleepiness Scale (KSS)

1. Extremely Alert
2. Very Alert
3. Alert
4. Rather Alert
5. Neither alert, nor sleepy
6. Some signs of sleepiness
7. Sleepy, but no effort to keep awake
8. Sleepy, some effort to keep awake
9. Very sleepy, great effort to keep awake—fighting sleep.

As the KSS takes less than a minute to complete, this contrasts with the much lengthier objective measures of sleepiness, seen with the PVT and MSLT, requiring, respectively, 10 minutes and up to 20 minutes duration, and thus able to detect a sleepiness that might be missed by the short duration subjective scales, or because of claims that we are apparently poor at assessing our own sleepiness, with which I disagree, for the following reasons.

Both the MSLT and PVT are insensitive to sleepiness if they were also to be given for only a minute, that is, for a duration comparable with that allowed for the KSS and similar scales. Moreover, detecting sleepiness using any of these methods depends not only on the test duration, but also on the degree of tedium that develops after one's self-motivated initial alertness wanes. Furthermore, the MSLT and PVT have the advantage of being given under quiet, non-distracting and relaxing settings, whereas this is often not the case with subjective measures, when the participant might have just sat down to complete the scale, and then moved to these other test settings. With these subjective measures there is usually insufficient time to settle down and relax before completing the scale, and certainly not enough time to let one's true feelings of sleepiness become apparent, as with the PVT for example. Remember, sleepiness feeds on boredom and monotony. We [12] have clearly shown that people are quite able to detect their own level of sleepiness if they are allowed five minutes or so to settle down and relax, which is a comparable period by which time the PVT usually begins to indicate sleepiness.

8.5   Mind over Matter

What people do and think about before and during all these tests is also critical to the outcome, as we and others have also shown on many occasions, with the PVT also being prone to these factors. In one of our studies [13] on the effects of boredom, healthy, non-sleep-deprived volunteers were quietly ushered into a lounge to wait alone for half an hour prior to undergoing the PVT. There were two conditions, one having the lounge containing dull and outdated technical magazines, with a TV showing a tedious video of how to grade potatoes. In the other condition there were interesting, topical magazines and amusing TV cartoons. Subsequently, there was a marked difference in the reaction time scores between the conditions, with many more lapses following the dull wait.

In another of our studies [14], using a more prolonged 30-minute PVT session during the mid-afternoon and with sleepy participants, two comparable groups were both given decaffeinated coffee. One was told that it was regular coffee with caffeine to keep them awake, and the other group was told that it was 'only decaffeinated coffee'. Performance was markedly better under the former condition, despite being caffeine-free.

On the other hand, if moderately sleepy people are told that they will receive an attractive monetary reward for avoiding lapses during a 10-minute PVT, then there are no lapses, unlike under the normal conditions [15]. However, by extending the PVT, here, to 30 minutes even the determination of the rewarded group to remain alert, fails towards the end, despite their best efforts to perform well.

Money can also influence the MSLT [16], as we have also seen with healthy, only moderately sleepy participants undergoing the usual MSLT, with half of them unexpectedly told that they will receive a financial reward for falling asleep as soon as they can. Accordingly, they get more comfortable, adopt their more idiosyncratic sleeping position, settle down more rapidly, fluff up the pillows and fall asleep around five minutes faster than when told nothing beyond the standard instruction of 'relax and try and go to sleep'.

Thus the attitude of the participant to the testing procedure is so very important, especially for the MSLT, as this test is often seen to be a 'physiological' and 'clinical' index of sleepiness, and especially as the EEG is also being measured, unlike the usual, seemingly more 'psychological' PVT. Yet, as the PVT is often also referred to as a 'neurobehavioural' measure of sleepiness, this also seems to make it more physiological and clinical. Nevertheless, apart from sleepiness, and as we have seen, both measures clearly show the influence of emotions, alertness and general 'state of mind'.

Of course, most good experimental studies of sleepiness fully appreciate all these extraneous variables, and are careful to adhere to strict, standard procedures. But even then participants can 'outwit' their experimenters, as we have seen ourselves with the PVT where, despite being undertaken in a small soundproof, visually sterile cubicle, designed to avoid all unwanted distractions, participants will even contrive 'games' to play in order to offset this tedium, such as making words out of the first row of the keyboard, working out the volume of the cubicle by counting the soundproof tiles, and by doing sums in their head. Such diversions, resulting in missed signals and the appearance of lapses, can be seen with non-sleep-deprived, alert but very bored individuals, who might thus be viewed to have 'hidden sleepiness' of which they were seemingly unaware, as they had reported subjectively, on the KSS, for example, that they were quite alert.

8.6   Twice as Sleepy or Half Alert?

Overall, and as I mentioned, the average MSLT score for normal sleepers is about 12–15 minutes. As those who do not fall asleep in a session are usually assigned a score of 20 minutes, in effect, this assumes that they might well have fallen asleep during the 21st minute had the test continued for another minute, thereby causing a 'ceiling effect' that skews these data. Various methods have been introduced to try and deal with this problem, but the real difficulty, here, is what exactly do these scores mean in terms of level of sleepiness? For example, 5-minute improvements in MSLT score from 5 to 10 minutes or from 10 to 15 minutes and from 15 to 20 minutes are numerically equal in terms of changes in sleepiness. But, put differently, someone with a MSLT of 5 minutes is apparently twice as sleepy as someone with a score of 10 minutes who in turn is twice as sleepy as someone with a MSLT of 20 minutes. However, there is no real basis on which to make this latter claim, and few would actually do so, but, in effect, this is how this linear (equidistant) time scale is used in statistical terms.

The same argument applies to the PVT, which also produces data on a linear scale, reflecting what is probably not a linear process—does a doubling of lapses indicate a doubling of sleepiness? And few would suggest that we could attribute 'twice as sleepy' in terms of a doubling of reaction times. A related issue mentioned in Sect. 6.5, is whether two nights of total sleep loss, compared to one night, will double sleepiness, irrespective of PVT or MSLT findings? Obviously, conceptualising sleepiness in this manner makes as little sense as would suggesting that hunger can be 'doubled' by going without two meals instead of one. Nevertheless, we do use the language of quantity to describe sleepiness, which is another reason why language based, subjective scales such as the KSS do have a key role to play and, in their own way, are just as important and meaningful as the objective measures.

There are some similar conundrums relating to sleepiness that can be illustrated by the MSLT. The first is based on the widely acknowledged average MSLT score being around 12–15 minutes for healthy, good sleeping adults. It implies that about half the healthy population will fall asleep faster than this, and suggests that a few minutes or so before falling asleep they would have been sleepy—sufficiently so to fall asleep. If they had felt alert prior to entering the MSLT bedroom, then this again shows that sleepiness can be 'unmasked', or maybe even generated in ostensibly alert people, if they so wish. Of course, it might be argued that this average MSLT latency includes a substantial proportion of the population with sleep debt, as they fail to attain a potentially desirable much longer MSLT score, indicative of what might be viewed as 'full alertness'. But there is probably little to be gained by asking the participant who has fallen asleep during the MSLT how sleepy they were prior to dropping off, as we know that falling asleep itself clouds such a judgement, as will be seen in the next section.

Another aspect of sleepiness, relating to the normal distribution of sleep and sleepiness, is as follows. If healthy, fully sleep-satiated people have their night sleep restricted by a fixed amount, either in absolute or proportional terms, then due to the normal distribution between people, some will naturally have shorter MSLT scores than others, despite the same sleep loss. Alternatively, if the normal sleep lengths for a variety of healthy sleepers of similar age and sex are ranked so that their MSLT scores are identical, then presumably there will be a normal distribution in these sleep durations. A similar finding may well be seen with other measures of sleepiness despite these constant MSLT scores. These various normal distributions may well belie more interesting interpretations, not only in terms of the relationships between sleep durations and MSLT scores in healthy good sleepers, but have wider implications.

In effect, this all means that for any given 'quantum of sleepiness' there is a normal distribution in the ability of healthy people to fall asleep. Whilst on the one hand, there will be those people who, naturally, will need a higher degree of sleepiness before falling asleep, on the other hand, and excluding those who are actually sleep deprived, there will be some, in this distribution, who can, if they so wish, fall asleep relatively rapidly but are not necessarily particularly sleepy, as was found in the study of those patients successfully treated for obstructive sleep apnoea (Sect. 8.2). This 'high sleepability', not so much due to sleep loss, is also seen by us and others [17, 18] in some healthy young adults having very short MSLT scores, below 6 minutes. To test whether they really were sleepy, we [16] gave them a much longer PVT session, lasting half an hour. But there were no lapses and their reaction times were normal—in fact better than normal. That is, they seemed quite able to decide whether or not to fall asleep, when in the appropriate circumstances.

8.7   Road Safety

With the possible exception of certain severe clinical conditions (e.g. narcolepsy), sleep does not occur spontaneously from an alert state. There is always a feeling of sleepiness beforehand, and apart from our findings clearly demonstrating this [19, 20] other research groups have also done so [21]. Thus, it is not possible to be alert one minute and asleep the next—certainly if one has no intention of falling asleep. This has important medico-legal implications for drivers who fall asleep at the wheel [22], who often claim that before the collision they had no feeling of sleepiness and thus fell asleep without forewarning. However, as we have seen, when given a few minutes to settle down, people have good insight into any sleepiness.

Somewhat paradoxically, and apart from sleep itself, sleepiness also clouds one's memory for recent sleepiness, as we have also found [17] when using a real car interactive road driving simulator, where drivers who had their EEG's recorded, with their faces monitored for eye closures, had to report their level of sleepiness (using the KSS) every few minutes during the drive. Although those having a microsleep at the wheel (seen in the EEG and by eye closure) are quite able to declare beforehand, that they feel sleepy, they cannot remember this actual feeling after the drive, despite remembering saying that they were sleepy. This phenomenon applies to all of us with, for example, our usual failing to remember, today, the actual feeling of sleepiness and how sleepy we were before bedtime last night and, particularly, when this became noticeable. The same applies to hunger and thirst—we can seldom remember either in any detail even a short while after a meal or drink, even though it was clear at the time that we were hungry or thirsty. The reason is that the human brain does not have the capacity to remember such pointless information after the consummatory acts of sleeping, eating and drinking.

Yet, sleepy drivers often reach a point of 'fighting sleep' revealed by their opening the car window (for fresh air), turning up the radio, stretching and so on, which must be self-evident that they are sleepy. Sleep is a dangerous state, and all living organisms are provided with behaviours necessary to ensure that they do not fall asleep spontaneously, and have forewarning to allow them to reach a place of relative safety. But the real problem, here, is that drivers will often continue to drive in this state, taking the risk in believing that they are able to remain awake, but are actually unable to predict if and when they will fall asleep. Of course, if someone is driving in the small hours of the morning, when they would usually be asleep in bed, and knowingly have had little sleep that night, then this is another reason why sleepiness would be self-evident.

In having fallen asleep, and then to know that one has been asleep, this sleep has to last at least a minute or so. Waking someone up who has momentarily 'dropped off' unexpectedly with an unscheduled sleep of less than this duration usually results in the sleeper's genuine disbelief of having been asleep. Sleepiness and the process of falling asleep clouds one's ability to know whether one is asleep or awake during this initial transition period. Which is a reason why most drivers who momentarily fall asleep for a few seconds at the wheel and have a collision subsequently have little recollection of actually having fallen asleep.

8.8   Circumspection

Sleepiness as a propensity to fall sleep and as an index of the 'biological need for sleep' are not necessarily synonymous, as its various measures reflect both essential and less or even non-essential aspects of sleep. That is, these measurement devices and their varying methodologies also encompass, to varying extents, different qualitative aspects of sleepiness apart from its intensity, that depend on, for want of a better term, 'the influence of the mind'. Besides, as neither sleep nor sleepiness seem to reflect uniform, equally proportional or numerically equivalent dimensions, then statistically significant outcomes can sometimes have less biological, psychological or clinical significance, or even obscure real sleep needs. Furthermore, the more sensitive a test of sleepiness is, especially in the laboratory environment, then the more it will be able to eke out the relatively inconsequential aspects of sleep and sleepiness. Thus, levels of sleepiness 'unmasked' in the laboratory by refined tests, but small enough to be unnoticed by healthy people leading normal lives in more stimulating environments, should make us circumspect in assuming these levels of sleepiness to be realistic, especially when these lead to claims of chronic 'sleep debt' in the general population. It is even possible that sleepiness can be generated *de novo* by a particularly dull and tedious situation. Nevertheless, I have argued that people do have good 'online' insight into their own sleepiness, whereas experimental findings indicating otherwise seem largely an artefact of the methodologies. Sleepiness is potentially life-threatening and for Nature not to have made provision for us to detect this in ourselves is most unlikely. The real danger for sleepy people is for them to 'consciously deny' their sleepiness and take sleepiness-related risks.

References

1. Lim, J, Dinges DF. 2008. Sleep deprivation and vigilant attention. *Ann N Y Acad Sci.* 1129, 305–322.
2. Van Dongen HP et al 2003 The cumulative cost of additional wakefulness: Dose-response effects on neurobehavioral functions and sleep physiology

from chronic sleep restriction and total sleep deprivation. *Sleep* 26, 117–126.

3. Littner MR et al 2005. Practice parameters for the clinical use of the MSLT and MWT. *Sleep*, 28: 113–121.

4. Geisler P et al 2006 The influence of age and sex on sleep latency in the MSLT 30- a normative study. Sleep, 29: 687–692.

5. Bonnet M & Arand DL 2001 Arousal components which differentiate the MWT from the MSLT. *Sleep* 24:441–447.

6. Sangal BB et al 1992 Maintenance of wakefulness test and multiple sleep latency test. Measurement of different abilities in patients with sleep disorders. Chest 101:898–902.

7. Engleman HM et al 1994. Effect of continuous positive airway pressure treatment on daytime function in sleep apnoea/hypopnoea syndrome. *Lancet.* 343: 572–575.

8. Dinges DF, Kribbs NB. 1991 Performing while sleepy: effects of experimentally induced sleepiness. in Monk, T.H. (ed) *Sleep, Sleepiness and Performance*; Winchester, John Wiley, Pp97–128.

9. Anderson C, Horne JA. 2006. Sleepiness enhances distraction during a monotonous task. *Sleep.* 29, 573–576.

10. Anderson C et al 2010. PVT lapses differ according to eyes open, closed, or looking away. *Sleep*, 33:197–204.

11. Åkerstedt T, Gillberg M. 1990 Subjective and objective sleepiness in the active individual. *Int J Neurosci* 52:29–37.

12. Horne JA, Burley C. 2010 We know when we are sleepy: subjective versus objective measurement of moderate sleepiness in healthy adults. *Biol Psychol* 83:266–288.

13. Mavjee V, Horne JA 1994 Boredom effects on sleepiness/alertness in the early afternoon vs early evening, and interactions with warm ambient temperature. *Br J Psychol* 85: 317–334.

14. Anderson C, Horne JA 2008 Placebo response to caffeine improves reaction time performance in sleepy people. *Human Psychopharm*, 23: 333–336.

15. Horne JA, Pettitt AN 1985 High incentive effects on vigilance performance during 72 h of sleep deprivation *Acta Psychologica* 58: 123–129.

16. Harrison Y et al 1996 Can normal subjects be motivated to fall asleep faster? *Physiol Behav*, 60: 681–684.

17. Lavie P, Zvuluni A. 1992. The 24 hour sleep propensity function: experimental bases for somnotypology. *Psychophysiol.* 29, 566–575.

18. Harrison Y, Horne JA 1996 High sleepability without sleepiness. *Clin Neurophysiol*, 26: 15–20.

19. Reyner LA, Horne JA 1998 Falling asleep at the wheel: are drivers aware of prior sleepiness? *Int J Legal Med* 111: 120–123.

20. Horne JA & Baulk SD 2003 Awareness of sleepiness when driving. *Psychophysiol*, 41: 161–165.

21. Åkerstedt T et al 2014 Subjective sleepiness is a sensitive indicator of insufficient sleep and impaired waking function *J Sleep Res*. 23:240–252.

22. Horne J, Rumbold J. 2015 Sleep related road collisions. *Med Sci Law*. 55: 183-185 .

9

Extreme Sleepiness

9.1 Badly Disrupted Sleep

Inadequate sleep comes in various forms. For example, it can just be too short, or at the wrong time of the day as in shift work, where both can produce excessive daytime sleepiness (EDS). Alternatively, this inadequacy can be more of a subjective state, as we have seen with insomnia, where the patient's distress is not so evident in objectively defined sleep when seen with overnight polysomnography (PSG) and absence of EDS.

During normal sleep we naturally move and change position, momentarily, about five times an hour, which usually necessitate short, 2–3 second, waking arousals. Such interruptions are unnoticeable and too short to cause any real sleep disturbance. However, when they become longer and more frequent, then this impaired sleep can become an even greater factor in determining waking well-being than can sleep duration, with the key sign usually being EDS, depending on the severity of the disruptions. For a sleeper to realise they have woken up during the night and to have remembered this next morning, they usually have to be actually awake for at least 30 seconds, more likely a minute or so, which is why short duration awakenings due to obstructive sleep apnoea (OSA) and

© The Editor(s) (if applicable) and The Author(s) 2016
J. Horne, *Sleeplessness*, DOI 10.1007/978-3-319-30572-1_9

periodic limb movement disorders of sleep (PLMD, see below) go unnoticed by the sleeper, despite occurring frequently during sleep. Sufferers are usually oblivious to their sleep having been so grossly disturbed, and may well believe that they have slept well. Such persistent daytime sleepiness, day after day, month after month, can reach such a chronic level that the patient 'forgets' what it is like to be normally alert, to the extent that they may well think this sleepiness is 'normal' for them. Treatments (mentioned below) can be remarkably effective and rapid, often dramatically noticeable to the patient, literally overnight, when they can wake up feeling sufficiently alert to realise how persistently sleepy they had really been.

Thus, inadequate sleep has marked contrasts, reflected by insomnia on the one hand, with its hyperarousal and perceived poor sleep, to OSA and PLMD, with both the latter usually accompanied by EDS and with the patient often unaware that their sleep is so poor. These latter two are the most prevalent sleep disorders in terms of severity of sleep disturbances and provide other important perspectives on sleep quality and sleepiness, which I will describe. The rarer narcolepsy-cataplexy will provide yet another perspective.

9.2   Excessive Daytime Sleepiness (EDS)

The most commonly used subjective scale for assessing EDS, is the Epworth Sleepiness Scale [1], which is self-explanatory:

The Epworth Sleepiness Scale (ESS)
How likely are you to doze off or fall asleep in the following situations, in contrast to just feeling sleepy?
    For each of the situations listed below give yourself a score of 0 to 3, where:
    0 = Would never doze
    1 = Slight chance
    2 = Moderate chance
    4 = High chance
Work out your total score by adding up the scores for situations 1–8.

If you have not been in one of these situations recently, think about how you might have been affected.

1. Sitting and reading
2. Watching TV
3. Sitting inactive in a public place (e.g. cinema, theatre, meeting)
4. As a passenger in a car for an hour without a break
5. Lying down to rest in the afternoon
6. Sitting and talking to someone
7. Sitting quietly after lunch (when you've had no alcohol)
8. In a car while stopped in traffic

TOTAL............
Conventionally, EDS is diagnosed when these scores total 11 and above.

9.3   Obstructive Sleep Apnoea (OSA)

OSA is the commonest form of severe sleep disruption, seen and heard by very heavy snoring. Patients with OSA can have no EDS, with ESS scores within the normal range, which suggests that the mechanisms underlying sleep cope with or adapt to this degree of sleep disturbance and, hence, symptoms are even more likely to go unnoticed by sufferers. This apparently milder OSA is not accompanied by the hyperarousal as happens with insomnia. However, when OSA reaches the point to cause EDS, then it is called 'OSA syndrome' (OSAS); that is 'syndrome', here, is synonymous with EDS.

The upper airway at the back of the throat is a rather flabby tube largely kept open by surrounding muscle tension, normally allowing the free flow of air in and out of the lungs when breathing during wakefulness. In sleep these muscles relax, and during inhalation this part of the airway, known as the 'oropharynx', sags inwards owing to the lower air pressure, as happens when breathing in. Too much of this 'flabbiness' leads to 'vibrations', which is, the more normal, mild snoring. Usually, we breathe through the nose during sleep, with mouth closed, thus clamping the tongue against the roof of the mouth to prevent it sagging back into the oropharynx, which would otherwise create even more obstruction and greater snoring. Snoring happens when the nose is partially blocked, necessitating mouth breathing, as can happen with, for example, a broken nose, a stuffy cold or hay fever. This snoring, like OSA, also usually goes unnoticed by the sleeper, unlike for those nearby whose sleep is often greatly affected. Depending on the anatomy of one's oropharynx, breathing through the mouth like this can cause total inward collapse of this upper airway, as seen with OSA. Other causes of OSA can be enlarged tonsils (especially in children), a small lower jaw, deformed palate, and an excess of folds in the mucous membrane that lie on either side of the oropharynx.

However, without doubt, the most common cause of OSA is obesity, particularly a fat neck, with a collar size greater than 17 inches (43 cm) in a man of average height. This, together with a large 'pot belly' and in men aged over 50 years predisposes them to OSA. Here, the additional weight of fat around the neck when lying asleep further compresses and thus collapses the oropharynx, with breathing further worsened by the 'pot belly' which can compromise the breathing actions of the diaphragm during sleep.

In each episode of OSA, the sleeper is gagged by the collapsed oropharynx, unable to breathe, even though the chest remains heaving in an attempt to suck air into the lungs. With falling blood oxygen levels ('desaturations') blood pressure rises, and the heart beats irregularly. Individual apnoeas can last for 10 seconds or longer, at which point breathing control centres in the brain respond by partially waking the individual, whereupon muscle tone within the oropharynx returns to normal, the airway opens up and there is a huge inrush of air, causing a series of very loud ('heroic') snores. After around 10–20 seconds, blood oxygen levels normalise and sleep returns, only for the whole cycle to be repeated, every few minutes. Sometimes, every minute, even more so in severe cases, and throughout much of sleep, or what is left of sleep, every night, month after month, maybe for years at a time.

Regardless of OSA or OSAS, and despite these persistent reductions in oxygen availability to the brain, called 'hypoxic episodes', the extent of cognitive impairment during wakefulness, apart from sleepiness, is not as great as might be expected, and everyday behaviour may well appear fairly normal, although there can be subtle changes with memory and within certain brain regions [2, 3]. This is not to dismiss the seriousness of OSA, but indicates whatever benefits sleep provides for the brain, its ability to cope with this continuous hypoxic onslaught, at least in the short term, is remarkable, as is the case for the heart and lungs, which are also under greater strain during these episodes. Eventually, though, and in more severe cases, OSA will at least worsen (if not cause) underlying cardiovascular disease, increase the risk of a stroke, and is likely to underlie what is known as drug resistant hypertension. However, the most life-threatening risk from OSAS comes from the EDS and a related accident.

During periods of OSA, the oropharynx might not always completely close, but breathing is still insufficient and blood oxygenation still falls, not quite to the full extent as that with total obstruction, and this state is called 'hypopnea'. The average number of apnoeas and hypopneas per hour of sleep, sufficient to cause blood oxygen desaturations usually greater than 5 %, and lasting for 10 or more seconds, together provide the apnoea-hypopnea index (AHI), indicating the severity of OSA. AHI is graded in averages per hour of sleep, as follows: Normal = 0–4; Mild Sleep Apnoea = 5–14; Moderate Sleep Apnoea = 15–29; Severe Sleep Apnoea = 30 or greater.

There is no effective drug treatment for OSA, whereas weight reduction, if obesity is the most likely cause, can produce an actual cure. However, as weight loss is easier said than done, then effective treatment for OSA is usually by 'continuous positive airway pressure' (CPAP). Here, room air at a slightly higher pressure, from a small pump, is supplied through a nose mask or, if nasal breathing is impaired, then a full mask is used. This air pressure dilates the oropharynx and allows for normal breathing. Ideally, CPAP should be used throughout the whole night, when it will usually stop OSA immediately. A less obtrusive and often just as effective alternative to CPAP, is a type of denture plate, worn during sleep, that pulls the lower jaw forward, thus opening up the back of the throat, allowing normal breathing. Both this and CPAP have to be fitted professionally.

There is another less common form of sleep apnoea known as central sleep apnoea, not caused by collapse of the upper airway, but due to the breathing control centre in the brain just switching off repeatedly during sleep. Usually, there is little sign of breathing (no chest movements or snoring) but, like OSA, the fall in blood oxygen level causes a momentarily awakening, when there is loud gasping with rapid and deep breathing, followed by a return to sleep as in OSA. Again, these awakenings are too short to be remembered but can be frequent enough to cause EDS. Unfortunately, CPAP is of no use, here, although drug treatment can help. In some cases central sleep apnoea can be triggered by OSA.

Too much alcohol in the evening can easily cause all three types of sleep-related breathing disorder concurrently, even in otherwise non-snorers. Not only does alcohol cause the oropharynx to further relax, even collapse to create OSA, but alcohol also causes hypopneas and central apnoeas. Not surprisingly, all contribute to that morning hangover.

9.4   Kicks and Restless Legs

Everyone has had that occasional sudden waking up 'with a jump', which is usually only a single kick of one or both lower legs. This is normal, unlike a form of PLMD known as nocturnal myoclonus or 'hypnic jerks', where this kicking is far worse, usually comprising a series of four or more successive kicks in rapid succession, lasting a few seconds, only to recur around every 30 seconds or so, not only at sleep onset, but often persisting well into sleep. It is a neurological disorder varying in the extent to which it disturbs sleep, from little to gross disturbance, with the latter causing EDS. Nevertheless, most of these episodes also go unnoticed by the sleeper, unlike that for the bed-partner receiving these kicks. Another form of PLMD, 'restless legs syndrome' often begins during evening wakefulness and, typically, is an unpleasant 'creeping-crawling' sensation within the thighs or calves, brought on by sitting or lying, but relieved by getting up and walking about. Hence, it is more noticeable to the patient than is nocturnal myoclonus. Low blood iron levels can cause both these types of PLMD, as can a build-up of urea in the blood, especially during pregnancy (disappearing after the birth). Apart from iron supplements for iron deficiency, treatments with 'dopamine agonists' in the evening to increase the brain's levels of the neurotransmitter 'dopamine' can rapidly be effective. I should add that PLMD is not necessarily confined to the legs as it can also affect one or both arms.

9.5   Narcolepsy

With this neurological ailment, which has the appearance of a disorder of REM sleep, there are daytime 'sleep attacks' lasting several minutes, preceded by sudden, overwhelming feelings of sleepiness. Here, REM sleep often appears soon after sleep onset. Narcolepsy is typically associated with 'cataplexy', usually separate from the sleep attacks, but also suddenly appearing during normal wakefulness, mostly triggered by surprise or excitement, including laughter. During cataplectic attacks, the sufferer remains awake but with what appears to be a REM sleep-like paralysis (see Sect. 13.1). This can result in a total collapse onto the floor, or be partial, only confined to the legs giving away, or just a sagging head. Full recovery is usually fairly quick, within a minute or so.

Narcolepsy-cataplexy has nothing to do with epilepsy, and usually becomes apparent during the teens. At least in part, it has a genetic basis, but may also have been triggered by an autoimmune response maybe following a viral infection. It is also accompanied by fragmented nighttime sleep, of which the sufferer is usually quite aware. Other symptoms include paralysis (sleep paralysis) at sleep onset and on morning awakening, lasting for a minute or so, often accompanied by sometimes frightening visual (hypnagogic) hallucinations, resembling waking dreams. Sodium oxybate is typically used to treat and suppress the cataplexy, and can also stabilise nighttime sleep, which in turn can help reduce the daytime sudden sleepiness and narcoleptic attacks. Psycho-stimulant medications, especially 'modafinil' (usually the drug of choice) can be particularly useful in suppressing this sleepiness.

References

1. Johns MW. 1991 A new method for measuring daytime sleepiness: The Epworth Sleepiness Scale. *Sleep* 14: 540–545.
2. Macey PM et al 2008 Brain structural changes in obstructive sleep apnea. *Sleep* 31:967–977.
3. Chen HL et al 2015 White matter damage and systemic inflammation in obstructive sleep apnea. *Sleep*, 38: 361–370.

10

Brainwork

10.1 Cortical Readiness

Sleep not only relieves sleepiness but has less obvious but equally vital functions for the cerebral cortex, which is the hardest working organ apart from exercising muscle. Even during relaxed wakefulness, with our eyes shut and the mind clear of thoughts, the cortex remains in a state of quiet readiness, ready to respond. Despite comprising only about 2 % of our body weight, it requires about 20 % of our oxygen consumption during wakefulness. Its largest area is the frontal lobe, occupying a third of the cortex (see Fig. 10.1). This region works even harder than the rest of the waking cortex, is at its most highly developed in us, and is the seat of what makes our behaviour uniquely human. Whereas 'sleepiness' is a phenomenon exhibited by all mammals, these sophisticated and largely subtle behaviours of ours, collectively called 'executive functions', are largely absent in rodents, for example, where their frontal cortex is poorly developed.

In wakefulness, none of the cortex can really recover from its workload or go 'offline', and only sleep, particularly SWS can provide for this. Moreover, SWS is at its most intense in this frontal region. On the other

J. Horne, *Sleeplessness*, DOI 10.1007/978-3-319-30572-1_10

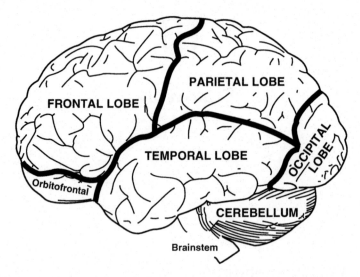

Fig. 10.1 Cortical lobes seen from the brain's left side. Note the large frontal lobe with its orbitofrontal region below

hand, the rest of the body can mostly recover during relaxed wakefulness, largely without needing sleep for its recovery. During sleep, especially during SWS (also reflected by Process S, Sect. 6.2) it is likely that synaptic and other interconnections between cortical neurones and glial cells (Sect. 10.4) undergo subtle modifications according their use during prior wakefulness.

All this is why a night without sleep is so evident in its impact on brain and behaviour, rather than on the functioning of other organs. However, most brain regions below the cortex do not seem to require sleep, including those involved in regulating vital body functions that have to continue throughout sleep, as well as those areas below the cortex that instigate and regulate more basic mechanisms of sleep itself.

10.2 Being Human

Despite the frontal cortex being largely responsible for our truly human behaviour, its significance in these respects was not realised until fairly recently, as neurologists, psychologists and others interested in brain function only utilised more routine, rather mechanistic tests that failed to tap into these subtle executive behaviours. In fact, many viewed the frontal area to be 'unnecessary' despite its large size, and the history behind this oversight provides for a fascinating account of how this aspect of medicine and neurology has evolved from being more of an art, formed of opinions and tradition, to a neuroscience based on exploration, discovery and wider insights. A historical account of this is given in the Appendix.

These executive functions include: focusing undivided attention onto something important, whilst ignoring competing distractions; deciding when to switch attention, often quite rapidly, as in 'multitasking'; comprehending and dealing with all types of novelty; coping with a rapidly changing situation, including knowing what to say in a changing and interactive conversation; updating plans following new information; remembering very recent events (working memory) and in what order they occurred; assessing risks, anticipating the range of consequences of an action; having insight into one's own performance; controlling ones 'uninhibited' behaviour (also associated with the orbitofrontal region, see Figs. 10.1 and 13.2); having empathy with other people, including detecting subtleties in their behaviour. In fact, all this is probably the source of consciousness as philosophers would define it, and of what Descartes perceived as, "*cogito ergo sum*" (I think therefore I am). In effect, without executive function we would be like automatons.

Even in modern psychological laboratories, these executive behaviours remain difficult to assess, as they are so different from reaction time tests and other simpler tests of sleepiness. Such behaviours are seldom seen under carefully controlled conditions where distractions and multitasking are minimised, and when spontaneous dialogues and other social interactions that would otherwise provide more clues, easily go unnoticed, especially during experimental studies of sleep loss. More about executive functioning and sleep in Chap. 11.

10.3 Brain Imaging

The waking demands on the cortex necessitate its large blood supply which not only provides oxygen, glucose and other nutrients, but removes waste products including the large amount of heat generated by all its activities. Functional magnetic resonance imaging (fMRI) of the brain enables three dimensional pictures to be constructed, every second or so, of localised blood flow that enable calculations then to be made (referred to as 'BOLD'—blood oxygen level dependence) of the localised oxygen utilisation, mostly by nerve cells. The greater this localised oxygen need, the greater nerve cell activity here. Although the level of this picture resolution is almost down to about one cubic millimetre (and improving), even this minute volume comprises thousands of cells. Thus, for the foreseeable future we do not have a comprehensive assessment of the actual activities within and around single or very small groups of brain cells, to see how they change activity during sleep compared with wakefulness.

Although changes to local blood flow and thus oxygen uptake can follow in less than a second after neural activity, this is a relatively long delay, considering that nerve impulses occur in a few tens of milliseconds. This time lag further adds to the considerable computing power needed to align more accurately oxygen uptake with presumed neural activity. Furthermore, as fMRIs comprise snapshots taken every second or so, several brain areas may 'light up' with each image, and so there is the problem of whether one area, and which one, came first, so as to unravel rapid 'chain reactions'. This is where the EEG can help, as it can be recorded continuously with fMRIs. But as the EEG from the scalp only detects what is going on towards the surface of the cortex, whereas fMRI goes deep down, then linking up these EEG changes with those of the fMRI again becomes rather problematic. Nevertheless, as many EEG electrodes (around 200) can be used to cover the scalp, the locations of the source of the various EEG waveforms emanating from different parts of the cortex can be identified. What is more, with this continuous EEG, the interactions over time between these waveforms and their locations can be calculated by, for example, 'nonlinear analysis', which is able to provide a reasonable method for tracing 'cause and effect' links in a chain of EEG events over very short periods of time, in milliseconds, and rather beyond the capability of fMRI. I will come back to this analysis, shortly, as it helps determine what parts of the cortex are, so to speak, really 'pulling the strings' during sleep as well as during wakefulness.

These issues further illustrate how far sleep science has to go in assessing what is really going on in the brain during sleep, and that investigators can be rather overwhelmed and even misled by impressive fMRI pictures. Similarly, we can perhaps all too easily correlate changes in localised fMRI and EEG activities during sleep with changes in certain behaviours the next day, even with aspects of waking memory, and assume a causal relationship. Of course, this is not to deny the impressive progress that continues to be made with all these techniques.

10.4 Glia: Silent Witnesses

We usually view the human cortex as comprising mainly nerve cells, but this is not so, as they are by far in the minority compared with glial cells ('neuroglia') that outnumber nerve cells by up to 20 to 1, depending whereabouts in the cortex, being at their most dense in the frontal lobes. The density of neuroglia to neurones is an index of behavioural complexity of a mammalian brain, and in the rodent cortex the ratio of neuroglia to neurones is mostly below 2:1, and for the chimpanzee it is up to 10:1.

Neuroglia have generally been overlooked as they are electrically silent compared with neurones, and have a lower oxygen need. The term 'neuroglia' comes from the Greek, meaning 'nerve glue' as these cells pack the spaces between neurones, and although they seem largely to nurture and protect neurones, we know relatively little about their functions compared with those of neurones. Yet the functions of neuroglia must not be underestimated as it is increasingly likely that they have many key roles, including as memory depositories.

Neuroglia come in different forms, having various names, such as 'astrocytes', which are not only intermediaries in supplying blood and nutrients to neurones (also largely forming the 'blood brain barrier'), but are almost certainly integral to information processing, as well as being able to 'talk' to each other in little understood ways. 'Microglia' can move around within the brain rather like amoeba, cleaning up debris and pathogens, as well as helping with the remodelling of synapses. In fact, some microglia are very much like white blood cells, able to 'squeeze' in and out of the walls of the brain's blood vessels and carry information about immunity between the brain and the rest of the body. Moreover, astrocytes and microglia produce substances called 'cytokines', able to induce and regulate sleep, although this is mainly during fever. Other neuroglia include 'oligodendrocytes' and 'Schwann' cells that form the insulating sheaths around the long axons of nerve cells, and can even stimulate the formation of synapses between neurones. Doubtless, neuroglia are probably as important as neurones to our understanding of what cortical recovery in sleep is all about.

10.5 'Hidden Attractor'

Despite my using 'SWS' (Stages 3 and 4 sleep) throughout this book so far, it is a loose term covering a rather arbitrary and relatively broad 'delta' EEG frequency range, from 0.5 to 3.5 Hz. Some years ago, the sleep pioneer, Professor Mircea Steriade, with colleagues [1] from the University of Montreal, identified a more specific and more interesting 'slow oscillation' of around 1 Hz (Fig. 10.2—lower) within the SWS

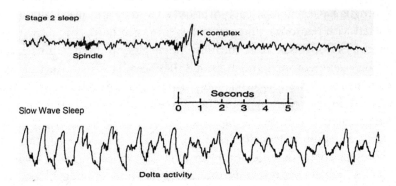

Fig. 10.2 Upper—Stage 2 sleep showing spindle and K Complex. Lower—1 Hz delta waves as seen in SWS. Note the similarity between these waves and the K Complex. See text for details

frequency range, which is probably more indicative of cortical reorganisation during sleep, especially in the frontal cortex, cf. [2], and where this 1 Hz activity is at its most intense compared with other cortical regions. Just now I mentioned 'nonlinear analysis', which is a technique mainly used in mathematical 'Chaos Theory' to determine the instigation and progress of a chain of events over short periods of time, as reflected by dynamic waveforms in complex systems, with the EEG being a good example. We [3] applied the method to this 1 Hz EEG, and found that not only was this EEG activity focused within the frontal area, to radiate over the rest of the cortex, but that this area seemed to be 'controlling' 1 Hz activity in these other cortical regions, to the extent that the frontal region seems to be the 'conductor' of cortical reorganisation during sleep. In Chaos Theory, the term used for this organiser, is 'hidden attractor'. Similarly, the frontal region is the 'hidden attractor' of our behaviour during wakefulness, as will be seen.

We [3] made two other interesting findings. First, this hidden attractor effect within the frontal area was most apparent during the first period of SWS, a finding that makes sense if sleep, especially SWS, and particularly 1 Hz, is critical for cortical recovery. Given that sleep is a vulnerable state, then its most important functions, especially this recovery, will no doubt be given priority. Second, this hidden attractor seems particularly oriented towards recruiting the parietal region of the cortex, and to a much greater extent in the sleep of healthy older people [3]. One explanation for this finding is that of the various cortical regions, it is the frontal area which declines the most in its abilities during normal ageing, maybe because it has worked the hardest for so long in one's lifetime. However, better news is that the frontal area seems to compensate for this by increasingly enlisting the parietal region as a back-up facility, seemingly with sleep and this 1 Hz activity playing an important role here, with the net result being much less of a deterioration in those waking behaviours relying on the frontal area. Remember, our cortex is unique in its continuing ability to adapt and learn throughout life, even old age, and is the topic of Chap. 12, as SWS, especially 1 Hz, also seems to be involved with this more major cortical reorganisation, as in 'use it or lose it' and thus contributes to a 'cortically healthy old age'.

Finally, a short note on the parietal area. It is largely involved in translating one sensation into another ('cross-modal transfer'). For example, in our being able to visualise an object in one's mind and physically identify it from hearing its name, but without having to see it, or in verbally naming or physically identifying an object by reading its name. These are just simple examples, and this area is also involved in our mental awareness of surrounding space and with the location objects, even knowing where our limbs and hands are ('body image') without looking at them. Interestingly, in backing up the frontal area, this parietal region seems able to handle in different ways certain of the 'executive' functions, covered more fully in the next chapter.

10.6 Stage 2 Sleep

Sleep research has paid much less attention to Stage 2 sleep (see hypnogram, Sect. 6.1) than it has to SWS and REM, as Stage 2 has been seen to be more as a 'filler' for sleep. Nevertheless, certain interesting EEG activities are prominent in Stage 2 (see Fig. 10.2—upper), with one being 'sleep spindles', otherwise known as 'sigma activity', and consisting of short, isolated bursts of 12–14 Hz waves, each usually lasting around a second, appearing about every 5–10 seconds. Spindles are also seen to a lesser extent in SWS. There are two types of spindle, a slower (12 Hz) variety coming from the frontal cortex, and a faster form (14 Hz) from the central 'sensorimotor' region of the cortex where the frontal and parietal lobes merge. This region deals with one's awareness of touch and conscious decisions about moving the trunk, limbs, fingers and so on, rather than the actual minutiae ('sub-routines') involved in the manipulation of individual muscles which are devolved 'down the line' to the cerebellum. Although fast spindles have been linked to procedural memory (see Sect. 10.7), this is still a speculative matter.

Stage 2 is a form of sleep defined by arbitrary cut-offs between the lighter Stage 1 sleep and SWS. Although it occupies almost half of our sleep, it is probably more of a dilute form of SWS [2] because its other prominent EEG characteristic, 'K Complexes', seem to be isolated 1 Hz waves (Fig. 10.2—upper). Like SWS, their appearance within Stage 2 declines during the course of sleep [2]. Interestingly, K Complexes in the latter part of sleep can be triggered by irrelevant sounds from the outside, and in this respect seem to protect the integrity of sleep [2], especially when they are accompanied by spindles. Thus, during a K Complex, as with SWS in its entirety, sleep is deeper and less able to be interrupted by wakefulness. Figure 10.2 (lower) shows a train of delta waves which are predominantly 1 Hz.

10.7 Memory

Apart from 'sleepiness', memory has been the focus of many recent studies interested in the functions of sleep, and various attempts have been made to see how sleep affects memory formation, including using fMRI and EEG methods. However, memory is a highly complex topic in itself, taking different forms, usually defined in terms of a hierarchy beginning with a simple division into short-term or working memory, lasting for less than a minute, and long-term memories that are enduring. I will just focus on long-term memory, which is further sub-divided into:

1. Implicit, unconscious memories, consisting of 'automatic' skills, such as playing a musical instrument or riding a bike, acquired through practice, so that we are no longer really aware of them. These are more commonly called 'procedural' memories.
2. Explicit or declarative memories, of which we are aware. These are further sub-divided into two types:

   (a) 'episodic memory', of events and experiences, e.g. encounters with things, places and people,
   (b) 'semantic memory' of facts and concepts, coming from reading, conversations, watching TV, listening to the radio, etc.

However, this usual categorisation is not all-encompassing, as there are also emotional memories, which may well involve REM, to be covered in Chap. 13.

During wakefulness, various different brain areas are involved with these types of memory, with certain areas particularly critical, these being the temporal lobe and its underlying hippocampus. Memories of whatever sort are mostly consolidated during wakefulness, with what seems to be a 'cleaning up' and some sort of integration within a 'bigger picture' undertaken during sleep. Nevertheless, given the duration of sleep, the extents to which various memories improve during sleep can be fairly small (albeit often statistically significant), at least from what can be determined from the typical test material used in memory research. Also somewhat debatable is the extent to which sleep is actively involved in positively improving memories, rather than just providing a period of reduced interference from the mass of incoming information from the senses, as happens during wakefulness.

However, most sleep and memory experiments consist of presenting some relatively simple material to be learned, just before sleep, followed by a period of sleep versus no sleep, then a retest. Usually, it is assumed that any such involvement of sleep will be confined to that immediate sleep rather than require a further sleep, maybe on a second night. For example, in studies of semantic memory, and the most common, the participant is given a series of word pairs to memorise, with only the first of the pair presented later, on retest, after sleep or nil sleep, with the participant having to recall its associated partner. A recent comprehensive review of these studies [4] concluded that the effect of sleep was only 'moderate' compared with just rest alone. Also, there are no consistent findings as to whether or what sleep EEG characteristics might reflect this particular memory processing, particularly as more than one sleep stage is implicated, although SWS is clearly critical.

While these memory tests are simple and rather unrealistic compared with what would be encountered in everyday life, one might well argue that sleep is more likely to be engaged with more sophisticated aspects of memory consolidation. Such as, integrating or abstracting this new information into wider concepts or knowledge having broader meanings, as has been proposed for sleep, more recently, cf. [5, 6]. Although these latter processes remain little explored, it is thought that aspects of SWS may well be critical here, cf. [5, 7].

In sum, and in terms of memory and sleep, we are only at the beginning of our understanding, and research has to be turned towards real-world and global aspects of what will invariably be very complex aspects of memory.

10.8 Lost Sleep

The frontal cortex is particularly vulnerable to total sleep loss because of its greater need for recovery, largely reflected by SWS and especially that 1 Hz activity. In broad terms, the effects on executive behaviours following a night without any sleep, and under real-world conditions, are seen as having difficulties in handling all forms of novelty, especially decision-making when there is uncertainty and distractions, more so when quick decisions are needed under unexpected circumstances. In contrast, during prolonged wakefulness, well-trained and highly skilled tasks, largely dependent on other cortical regions, seem less vulnerable to such sleep loss [8–12]. Consequently, during this sleep deprivation people will tend to revert to these latter skills, and in doing so become more rule-bound, rather than thinking more innovatively. Surprisingly, 'IQ type' tests are fairly resilient to sleep loss, being more logical, with all the possible answers and options to a problem being available, and it is just a matter of deduction and homing in on which is correct. However, with executive, innovative thinking and decision-making there are no obvious solutions, often false trails and irrelevant information, requiring one to 'think out of the box'.

Of course, the frontal region is also intimately involved in our 'conscious decisions' whether or not to go to sleep, despite circadian influences and 'Process C'.

Hence, it is important to study these effects of sleep loss under as realistic situations as possible, and although many psychological tests are claimed to be measuring executive function, this is often only partly so [12], as they are given under those dull, strictly controlled laboratory conditions without distractions. Besides, if used repeatedly these tests lose their novelty, as people acquire techniques or 'tricks' to deal with them, and so the test becomes 'automatic', and no longer a measure of executive function [9, 12]. That is, such tests are often too remote from the real world, and not sufficiently 'ecological'.

References

1. Amzica F, Steriade M. 1998 Electrophysiological correlates of sleep delta waves. *Electroencephalogr Clin Neurophysiol.* 107:69–83.
2. Halàsz P et al. 2014 Two features of sleep slow waves: homeostatic and reactive aspects. *Sleep Med*, 15: 1184–1195.
3. Terry JR, Anderson C, Horne JA 2004 Nonlinear analysis of EEG during NREM sleep reveals changes in functional connectivity due to natural aging. Hum Brain Mapping; 23:73–84.
4. Chatburn A et al 2014 Complex memory processing and sleep: a systematic review and meta-analysis of behavioural evidence and underlying EEG mechanisms. *Neurosci Biobehav Rev*;47C: 646–655.
5. Diekelmann S, Born, J. 2010, The memory function of sleep. Nature Rev Neurosci 11: 114–126.
6. Lewis PA, Durrant SJ. 2011 Overlapping memory replay during sleep builds cognitive schemata. *Trends Cogn Sci.* 15:343–351.
7. Cairney SA et al 2015 Complementary roles of slow-wave sleep and rapid eye movement sleep in emotional memory consolidation. *Cereb Cortex.* 25: 1565–1575.
8. Drummond SP et al 2004 Increasing task difficulty facilitates the cerebral compensatory response to total sleep deprivation. Sleep 27: 445–451.
9. Harrison Y, Horne 2000 The impact of sleep deprivation on decision making: a review. *J Exp Psychol Appl.* 6:236–249.
10. Maddox WT et al 2009 The effects of sleep deprivation on information-integration categorization performance. *Sleep* 31, 1439–1448.
11. Horne JA 2012 Working through the night- subtle impairments to critical decision making. Neurosci Biobehav Rev 36: 226–233.
12. Horne JA 2012 Testing of executive function. *Chronobiol Internat* 29:1284.

11

Prolonged Wakefulness

11.1 Night Work

Human errors in the early morning have been implicated in preventable disasters, such as those with the Three Mile Island and Chernobyl nuclear reactors, and the loss of the space shuttle 'Challenger' [1]. In all cases, operators had been awake for almost 24 hours and failed to correctly diagnose a problem, then adopted a wrong course of action and persisted with it, unable to recognise the importance of new information requiring a change of plan. Obviously these disasters were not solely through failures of executive functions as psychological stress must clearly have been involved to compound matters but, nevertheless, these effects are symptomatic of 'executive' failures. Despite the Presidential Report on the Challenger disaster noting that, *"working excessive hours, while admirable, raises serious questions when it jeopardises job performance, particularly when critical management decisions are at stake"* [1], and the subsequent endeavours by various organisations to deal with these issues, little has really changed today, thirty or so years later. Night shifts have mostly increased from 8 to 12 hours, with critical decision-makers on their first night of a night shift, often having been awake for up to

© The Editor(s) (if applicable) and The Author(s) 2016
J. Horne, *Sleeplessness*, DOI 10.1007/978-3-319-30572-1_11

24 hours since their previous morning's sleep. On the second night, after some daytime sleep (see Sect. 7.5) this situation is eased.

Members of the medical profession undergoing similar night shifts, with little or no sleep, continue to be susceptible, being more likely to make a variety of diagnostic errors [2] especially when presented with a patient displaying an unusual variety of symptoms. Here, the sleep-deprived physician is more likely to focus unduly only on some symptoms, to the exclusion of others that might increasingly become of greater relevance. Having made a diagnosis he or she is more likely to persevere with it, despite otherwise obvious contraindications, and even argue unduly with colleagues whose opinions differ, as social interactions may well be compromised. Whilst coffee and other caffeinated drinks will help overcome sleepiness, they are less likely to counteract these executive impairments.

Other professions involving periods of prolonged night work without sleep and likely to encounter similar scenarios are seen with the military, the emergency services, and even '24/7 financial traders' having to deal quickly with fluctuating international markets. Usually, most of these situations requiring critical decisions can be foreseen and effectively resolved, with staff having been adequately trained and well prepared for a variety of eventualities. However, in the absence of prepared action plans, and having to deal with unforeseen, uncertain and rapidly changing events, requiring quick decisions, people under these sleep-deprived situations are less able to grasp and continue to update 'the big picture' and less likely to successfully 'fly by the seat of one's pants'. As well as difficulty in maintaining focus on key issues, keeping track of and remembering very recent developments, identifying and ignoring conflicting and irrelevant information, also affected is the ability to foresee and weigh up potential outcomes from a variety of possible decisions, and to be innovative in planning appropriate responses, cf. [3, 4]. Perseveration, that is persisting with an action that is increasingly pointless and losing one's insight into when to stop and direct attention elsewhere, becomes evident [3] and, for example, with undue fixations on irrelevant distractions. All of which have important implications for the real world.

Speech also becomes less articulate, 'flattened', more laboured and with longer pauses [3, 5]. Spontaneous dialogue becomes less interactive, fewer appropriate words come to mind, with shorter sentences and we rely more on clichés. There is more mumbling and mispronunciations, with slurring or words run together or in the wrong sequence.

Mood will often alter during a prolonged sleepless night, not just because of greater 'irritability' caused by general sleepiness, but because executive function also includes the ability to 'keep a cool head' in weighing up the relative risks and consequences for alternative actions, and not to overreact. Normally, the frontal cortex dampens down more excitable behaviours, making us more conventional, and socially aware of how others see us. Thus, one's perception of risk can become increasingly irrational. On the one hand, if people believe that they are likely to succeed in their actions, then they can become more optimistic, take greater risks and be more impulsive, sometimes even euphoric, especially in the early morning hours. That is, self-insight into how well one is working also deteriorates, as we think we are performing better than is usually the case, which could underlie why casinos are open throughout the night! On the other hand, perceived uncertainty as well as the physical and social circumstances will also influence decision-making and, for example, if one is alone and thinking of possible failure, then one becomes more 'risk averse' [4, 6].

Interestingly, the link between sleep and mood is most evident in those people suffering from severe depression, when a night of sleep deprivation can produce a marked lifting of the depression, only to lapse with recovery sleep. Moreover, for those suffering from periodic mania, these episodes are portended by little sleep the night before its occurrence, with sleep continuing like this, often for several weeks, until the mania subsides.

11.2 'Distractability'

While losing track of events during multitasking is worsened by prolonged wakefulness, largely due to a failure to recognise what actually mattes and ought to be attended to, at the other extreme, when the task is mundane and tedious we seek stimulation, that is, distractions, in order to try and stay awake, with perseveration affecting both these contrasting scenarios. In the case of the PVT, I described (Sect. 8.3) how distractions can cause signals to be missed, to resemble microsleeps, despite the test being performed under bland conditions, ostensibly with minimal distractions. Nevertheless, participants can still contrive distractions, which are usually longer than just a quick 'glance away', often owing to perseveration. This is a particular problem with 'drowsy driving' on monotonous roads (Sect. 8.7), when drivers are not only more likely to be distracted away from maintaining attention to the road, but perseverate with this for longer [7], thus heightening the likelihood of an accident.

In a realistic simulation of security screening, we undertook [8] an all-night replication of a first night on a night shift, with paid and trained operators who had been awake for over 20 hours. They watched a screen showing a continuous flow of moving X-ray images of luggage containing a variety of harmless personal belongings, that occasionally contained dummy weapons embedded within this distracting 'clutter'. In comparison with non-sleep-deprived operators, and even with inspection periods only lasting 30 minutes, those who were sleep deprived became progressively more distracted by this 'clutter' and missed some crucial items, whereas this did not occur with the other group. Of course, had this been for real, then they may well have performed better, although, they were well rewarded, here, and exhorted to do their best.

Outside the field of sleepiness and sleep loss, visual distraction by movement or movement-like activities (e.g. flashing light) in the visual periphery causes healthy, alert individuals looking ahead, to divert their gaze towards such movement. This is a well-known eye movement reflex, and the degree to which one can suppress this movement, known as an 'anti-saccade', largely depends on the integrity of part of the frontal cortex known as the 'frontal eye fields'. Whilst nothing is yet known about whether this suppression is affected by sleepiness, clinical findings outside the topic of sleep show that impairment to frontal lobe function interferes with these anti-saccades.

In sum, for whatever reasons, prolonged wakefulness decreases one's resistance to distraction, and that distraction itself, including perseveration with this distraction, are important aspects of sleep loss that require much more investigation.

11.3 Negotiations

Even with situations involving delicate discussions in the small hours, as with sleepless politicians trying to resolve deadlocks and negotiate terms, other aspects of executive function can be affected [3], where it has been shown that *"even a single night of total sleep deprivation can have dramatic effects on economic decision making"* [9]. Negotiators may well become more obdurate, likely to be sidelined by irrelevancies, lose track of when and what was recently said [3, 10], have difficulty in finding the appropriate (and diplomatic) words with which to express themselves [5, 10, 11], become more distrustful and wary of possible exploitation [12] and are less likely to detect in other people any subtle changes to their facial expressions and to non-verbal cues into how these people perceive the ongoing situation [11]. Furthermore, one is less able to track and update the underlying meaning in a conversation and, instead, be more liable to misconstrue another person's perspective, especially if it differs from one's own and thus one's potential ability to negotiate [11–16].

11.4 Countermeasures

With all these effects of prolonged wakefulness, and when unusual crises occur in the early hours of the morning, it is important that frontline decision-makers are aware of their potential shortcomings in these respects, and that this is not necessarily a poor reflection on them personally, but is where teamwork counts. Attitudes such as, 'it's my watch and I'll see it through', are laudable but inadvisable, especially when there are additional stresses. One can only wonder to what extent fateful military decisions have been made by sleep-deprived military commanders who have thus become overconfident, ill-tempered with their junior officers, and who failed to appreciate unexpected changes in enemy tactics and pressed on with what turns out to be a disastrous offensive.

I mentioned just now that caffeine and other stimulants cannot be relied upon as effective countermeasures to this form of impaired decision-making during marked sleep loss [3, 15]. However, in an emergency, even

3 hours sleep (allowing for some cortical recovery facilitated by SWS) followed by caffeine on awakening will certainly be worthwhile, although there is the problem of grogginess and sleep inertia.

11.5 Inertia

Finally, to pursue this military theme, and still with executive behaviours in mind, a sudden, unexpected awakening from early on in a night's sleep, especially from SWS, usually requires about 15 minutes or so for the frontal cortex to fully 'wake up' and become completely engaged with reality. This form of inertia is especially evident in young adults who normally have more intense SWS. We [17] ran an army exercise with 20 highly motivated junior officer reservists, each commanding a platoon of soldiers. Without any prior warnings, half the group were suddenly awoken at 3 a.m. after 2–3 hours' sleep and confronted with a simulated enemy attack. After a one-minute group briefing, each commander was separately presented with this scenario in the form of written details about the situation, with a significant portion of this information being quite irrelevant, with some of it purposely misleading. A detailed map was provided, showing both important and strategically useless landmarks, the likely 'enemy' position, and a list of available equipment and other support. The map had a relatively obvious 'best' route to take for a counterattack. Relevant information had to be extracted from this material, and under time pressure, as only 15 minutes was allowed for them to complete briefly written orders for their troops. However, after 10 minutes, when the plan should have been near to completion, and with each commander working on the finer details, they were (again unexpectedly) presented with an update on the situation, that should have made clear that the more 'obvious route' was now too dangerous and thus a new tactic was required. It told of sudden flooding due to previously persistent heavy rain, causing the loss of a vital footbridge, and the unexpected exposure of a hitherto unknown minefield, as well as a change in wind direction which would affect the use of smoke cover.

The other (control) group slept until 7.30 a.m. in a separate building. An hour later, having had adequate sleep and sufficient time to get up and begin a normal waking day, they were presented with the identical sudden emergency, again unexpectedly. Performance of all the commanders, from both situations, was scored under five categories, with three having executive behaviour themes. Scoring was by army instructors who had to judge the final written orders, seen randomly and without their knowing the group origins. Eight of the 'inertia' group versus three of the controls failed overall, with five of the former group, versus none of the latter making catastrophic errors. Three of this five were unable to change their plans, and adhered to the 'best route' (which would have resulted in 'wipe-out'), and two others wrongly repositioned their troops in hazardous areas. Other mistakes of an executive nature, clearly evident in the sleep inertia group, were poor risk assessment in being unable to appreciate a change in the wind direction when 'placing smoke', and a failure to avoid a change in the enemy position, situations that all the control group recognised. Also adversely affected (due to the loss of the footbridge) was the ability to quickly reassess the relevant from the irrelevant information, and determine the appropriate 'use of cover' (concealment), where previously identified (but now useless) cover continued to be adhered to, and new potential cover was overlooked. However, other logical and highly trained basic skills involving more rational thinking remained unimpaired in the experimental group. Examples of this were 'tactical awareness', involving appreciation of the usefulness of geographical features, and the capability of various items of weaponry.

Of course, this exercise was a 'worst-case scenario', and apart from this sleep inertia, the experimental group differed from the controls in having shortened sleep, and an earlier time of testing (within the circadian trough), all of which would have combined to clearly differentiate the two groups. And it was also a stressful situation for both groups. Needless to say, it was quite unlike more typical laboratory studies tending only to manipulate one of these three experimental variables at a time. Although this might be seen as too uncontrolled a study, it was relevant to real-life situations and involved highly motivated individuals requiring skills usually well within their capabilities, as they had received extensive military training and experience of real exercises.

Although ours was a simulation, the findings indicate that in comparable situations elsewhere, in the emergency services, for example, where one has to assimilate novel and unexpected events which then change, people should be mindful of these potential albeit temporary impairments to their flexible thinking ability, if and when suddenly awoken, early morning. Whilst it is possible that older people would not be so susceptible to sleep inertia, given that their sleep contains less SWS and is thus not so deep, this potential age difference remains unexplored. Ideally, older 'line managers', who are also likely to be more experienced, ought to be consulted before final decisions are made under these exacting circumstances, but this is not always feasible. Maybe all this helps explain why the military has such a predilection to 'attack at dawn' whilst the enemy is still asleep and could be caught unawares?

11.6 Summing Up

Sleepiness feeds on monotony, with the most sensitive laboratory tests of sleepiness maximising such tedium by making tests simple, dull and monotonous. However, this adverse effect can be counteracted to a marked extent by applying more mental effort, or by a stimulant such as caffeine. Such compensatory effort is implicit with more complex, stimulating, well-trained, logical and deductive tasks not so reliant on the frontal cortex, and thus not so affected by sleep loss, at least initially. On the other hand, more subtle and demanding 'executive' behaviours, largely depending on the frontal region are still vulnerable even when more effort is applied and caffeine is taken. This deteriorating executive function is evident even during a night of prolonged wakefulness, more so outside the laboratory under more real-world conditions.

With more prolonged sleep deprivation we become more like automatons, creatures of routine, losing spontaneity, less able effectively to deal with anything new and less aware of where to direct our attention or what to ignore, and displaying dull and stilted speech. We become more irritable, less able to suppress basic emotions or to 'sense' the feelings of others and detect nuances in their behaviour. Similar, albeit temporary effects can be seen when we are suddenly awoken from deep sleep, as the frontal area can take upto 20 minutes to become 'really awake' and fully engage with reality.

As SWS, more likely its 1 Hz component, seems to be critical to frontal lobe recovery, this means that a shortened sleep which allows for adequate SWS is less likely to have such a detrimental effect on executive function, and that residual sleepiness and adverse effects on simple monotonous tasks seem able to be largely overcome by caffeine, for example. Moreover, it is unlikely that those sufferers from insomnia, given that they do obtain this more vital sleep, will have impaired executive function.

Finally, a reminder that in the Appendix is a historical account of how science and medicine had overlooked the role of the frontal cortex, even until the late 1950s. The account also illustrates how investigators then, and even now, can be reluctant to break away from more traditional approaches and beliefs, which might otherwise risk research funding, the publication of such apparently 'anomalous' findings, even incur restraint by one's superiors or institutions whose reputations have to be maintained. It is so important for us to remain critical observers, able to note and question the unexpected and unusual, and to maintain at least some scepticism over outcomes especially when using standard methods and techniques.

References

1. NASA 1986 *Report of the Presidential Commission on the Space Shuttle Challenger Accident* http://science.ksc.nasa.gov/shuttle/missions/51-l/docs/rogers-commission/table-of-contents.html
2. Rothschild JM et al 2009. Risks of complications by attending physicians after performing nighttime procedures *J Amer Med Assoc* 302:1565–1572.
3. Horne JA 2012 Working through the night- subtle impairments to critical decision making. Neurosci Biobehav Rev 36: 226–233.
4. Killgore, W.D. 2010 Effects of sleep deprivation on cognition. *Prog. Brain Res.* 185: 105–129.
5. Harrison Y, Horne JA, 1997. Sleep deprivation affects speech. *Sleep* 20: 871–877.
6. Anderson C, Dickinson DL, 2010. Bargaining and trust: the effects of 36-h total sleep deprivation on socially interactive decisions. *J Sleep Res.* 19: 54–63.

7. Anderson C & Horne JA 2013. Driving drowsy also worsens driver distraction. *Sleep Med.* 14: 466–468.

8. Wales AW et al 2009 Evaluating the two-component inspection model in a simplified luggage search task.luggage search task. Behav Res Methods, 41; 937–943.

9. Libedinsky C et al 2011 Sleep deprivation biases the neural mechanisms underlying economic preferences *Front. Behav. Neurosci.*5, 70. Epub

10. Harrison Y, Espelid E. 2004 Loss of negative priming following sleep deprivation. *Quart. J. Exper. Psychol.* 57A: 437–446.

11. Harrison Y, Horne JA. 1998 Sleep loss impairs short and novel language tasks having a prefrontal focus *J. Sleep Res.* 7: 95–100.

12. McKenna BS et al 2007 The effects of one night of sleep deprivation on known-risk and ambiguous-risk decisions J. Sleep Res. 16, 245–245.

13. Pilcher JJ et al 2011 The effects of extended work under sleep deprivation conditions on team-based performance. *Ergonomics.* 54: 587–596.

14. van der Helm E et al 2010 Sleep deprivation impairs the accurate recognition of human emotions. *Sleep* 33, 335–342.

15. Ybarra O, Winkielman P. 2012 On-line social interactions and executive functions. *Front. Hum. Neurosci.* 6:75. doi: 10.3389/fnhum.2012.00075

16. Harrison Y & Horne JA 2000. Sleep loss and temporal memory. Quart J Applied Psychol. 53A: 271–278.

17. Horne JA. Moseley R. 2011. Suddden awakeningfrom curtailed night's sleep impairstactical planning in a realistic and changing 'emergency' scenario. *J Sleep Res* 20: 275–279.

12

Use It or Lose It

Few people know how to take a walk. The qualifications are endurance, plain clothes, old shoes, an eye for nature, good humour, vast curiosity, good speech, good silence and nothing too much.

Ralph Waldo Emerson 1803-1882

12.1 Enrichment

Engaging oneself in a stimulating, novel and varied environment increases the workload on the cortex and its 'brainwork', which leads to a greater need for cortical recovery and its 'plastic' or 'rewiring' processes during sleep, and largely reflected by SWS, cf. [1]. Moreover, in terms of waking 'use it or lose it', daily cortical 'workouts' to increase brainwork may well slow up the natural ageing of the cortex, particularly apparent in the frontal cortex, as I mentioned earlier (Sect. 11.5).

Heightened brainwork comes from just 'getting out and about' [1, 2], more so when this involves curiosity and exploration. That is, looking around and assimilating what is going on, then thinking and associating this information with past memories and emotions, and deciding what to do next, especially if this involves walking which brings new encounters and situations beyond normal routine. As we humans are so reliant on sight, more than any other sense, it provides the bulk of incoming information into the brain. Such brainwork can be quite pleasant, as in window shopping, visiting an exhibition or museum, sightseeing, going on holiday or enjoying the walk that Emerson describes. Socialising,

© The Editor(s) (if applicable) and The Author(s) 2016
J. Horne, *Sleeplessness*, DOI 10.1007/978-3-319-30572-1_12

engaging in conversations and meeting new people in the process further add to the novelty. This is what, for the cortex, a busy waking life is all about—engaging one's brain with interesting, absorbing and changing novelty. More to the point this will increase the amount of SWS, cf. [2], unlike staying indoors surrounded by familiarity and reading, viewing TV or an exciting film, even studying for an exam or doing a crossword or sudoku. These are not so effective, only really engaging smaller cortical areas and are relatively more passive activities compared with the 'full frontal demands' of this getting out and about.

Physical activity, especially walking, is integral to this brainwork, in telling the brain that more cognitive demands are probably on the way. Thus, cognition is almost inseparable from physical activity [2–4], and within the context of human ageing both processes are intrinsically linked to each other to increase cortical plasticity [4]. In sum, an enriched environment combined with physical activity and challenging cognitive tasks are the basis for potential interventions to promoting successful cortical ageing. Moreover, it seems that SWS, or at least its 1 Hz component (Sect. 10.5) reflects these beneficial processes.

12.2 Exercise Is Not Enough

Unquestionably, exercise has marked benefits for more general aspects of physical health and is often claimed to help delay the brain's natural ageing processes. However, in relation to the brain's 'use it or lose it', any multisensory stimulation, curiosity and cognitive load accompanying the exercise almost certainly plays a more crucial role than exercise alone. Whereas exercise and physical activity are a necessary 'vehicle' for this varied stimulation, walking on a treadmill in a featureless room, going nowhere, is not providing the brain with its workout. Even jogging outdoors, head down, staring at the ground, listening to an iPod and periodically grimacing at one's stopwatch, is too mundane in these respects.

The 'getting out and about' aspect of physical activity is largely overlooked by those advocating the benefits of exercise for the brain, and although recent reviews of this field, e.g. [5], find significant effects of exercise in preventing cognitive decline in the older person, these make little mention of the accompanying 'cognitive load', but instead tend to attribute the effect largely to improvements with the brain's blood supply and aspects of the brain's chemistry. However, at least one recent major review of this area [6] has been much more guarded about why some cognitive functions improve with exercise while others are insensitive. For example, although a year-long indoor walking programme in healthy older adults [7] pointed to (working) memory improvements, and to better physical fitness, there were no improvements to be seen with measures of executive function. Here, walking was monotonous, on an indoor circular track and, interestingly, it was noted [7] that with more environmental stimulation, these improvements may well have been greater.

Apparent benefits for the brain of exercise alone, usually soon disappear when the regimen is ended [8] and exercise taken to excess can be counterproductive, as the brain goes into a protective mode [9] that can be interpreted as a sign of improving brain health, which is not necessarily the case. On the other hand, brisk walking regimens and jogging can improve sleep quality and subjectively determined sleep in poor sleepers [10].

Despite physical exercise alone seeming to be able to reverse some detrimental effects of ageing on those aspects of memory that focus on the hippocampus [11] (Sect. 10.7), the same benefits are seen with a variety of non-exercise 'cognitive stimulations' [11] in normal healthy individuals, in particular, those activities involving novel experiences undertaken daily over several weeks as, for example, in taxi drivers learning new routes [12], with these improvements maintained for several months after training. Although healthy older people usually show obvious associations between their levels of physical fitness and cognitive function, including executive skills, all of this usually comes with a more mentally and physically active and outgoing lifestyle as well as with a positive attitude to one's life.

12.3 Boosting SWS

Sleep, particularly SWS and 1 Hz EEG activities, indicates the enhancing of brain plasticity [13], and these activities, and probably other (yet to be determined) aspects of the sleep EEG, can provide useful markers of the effects of this increased brainwork in terms of 'use it or lose it' for the ageing brain. However, more needs to be known about how long-term daily regimens of cognitive stimulation with and without accompanying physical exercise compare with each other. To date, such findings have been incidental as, for example, seen with a major study [14] of age-related cognitive decline linked to structural changes within the frontal cortex, and accompanied by diminished SWS. The investigators concluded [14] that these findings could be improved by behavioural interventions. Moreover, there is evidence [15] that three hours of daily structured but engaging social and physical activity in healthy elderly people leads to increased SWS, with improvements to memory-oriented tasks. However, this intervention [15] only lasted for two weeks, and it is not clear what would happen if this and similar activities were to be continued in the long term.

Interestingly, we [16] have found that older people who naturally and habitually have more SWS are more flexible in their thinking, have better executive skills, and thus seem to have a 'younger brain' for their age.

But simply using what might be viewed as more artificial methods to increase SWS in the sleep of the older person, is not necessarily a good sign of a more active waking brain, unless there is evidence of cognitive improvement. Certain drugs can also elevate SWS, as can short-term increases in waking brain temperature (thus increasing the brain's metabolic rate) but without any improvements to waking behaviour, cf. [2]. Nevertheless, a 30-minute warm bath in the evening, to increase both body and brain temperature not only increases SWS that night, but generally improves nighttime sleep in those healthy elderly with insomnia [17].

Of course, getting out and about, outdoors, and encountering daylight, will help synchronise the circadian clock and the timing of sleep, as well as have a daytime alerting effect and reduce the extent of daytime naps and thus promote better nighttime sleep.

Finally, increased levels of ß-amyloid in the cortex are associated with dementia. There is new evidence [18] that in older people these levels in areas of the prefrontal cortex are correlated with diminished amounts of SWS, especially its 1 Hz component, as well as with impaired hippocampus-dependent memory consolidation. However the extent to which there is any cause and effect, here, remains a matter for speculation, as might the benefits of the 'getting out and about' enhancement of SWS in older age have in offsetting progression of this ß-amyloid. But clearly this is a potentially worthwhile area of further investigation.

12.4 'Fresh Air'

Much can be said for the Victorian belief that exercise should be relaxing and not taxing, as advocated, for example by the pronouncements in 1900 by Dr James Sawyer in his article, *"Causes and Cure of Insomnia"*, published in the British Medical Journal (8 December 1900, p. 627) that, *"Daily bodily exercise in the open air but always short of great fatigue must be enjoined. What is called carriage exercise is better than no outdoor change at all, but walking is far better exercise and cycling better still, and riding on horseback the best of all. A worn and worrying man habitually wrapt up in an absorbing torture of self-consciousness and sleeping badly, must come out of himself with the saving graces when he mounts a cycle or horse's back."* And finally, *"Gardening in the open air, not in conservatories or hothouses affords good exercises and it is very efficient in keeping up objective attention."* As sleeplessness-cum-insomnia was generally thought at the time to be a problem for those with more cultured and educated minds, one must sympathise for the horseless, poor worker whose 'gardening' comprised struggling to grow a few vegetables in a meagre plot of land, so as to supplement the family's food supply.

We might smile at this naivety and that 'gardening makes good sport' but, nevertheless, these words of Dr Sawyer are wiser than they may seem, as not only does all this outdoor activity also expose one to daylight, but varied and active gardening will indeed 'exercise the brain', to create more brainwork, and in doing so may further improve sleep and SWS. Hence, many of us need to be more 'ecological' with our sleep and wakefulness, get out and about more, even commune with nature, take more of those relaxing baths, contemplate the wisdom of Emerson, and maybe cancel that subscription to the gym.

References

1. Halàsz P et al. 2014 Two features of sleep slow waves: homeostatic and reactive aspects. *Sleep Med*, 15: 1184–1195.
2. Horne JA 2013 Exercise benefits for the aging brain depend on the accompanying cognitive load: insights from sleep electroencephalogram. *Sleep Med* 14:1208–1213.
3. Fabel K, Kempermann G. 2008 Physical activity and the regulation of neurogenesis in the adult and aging brain. *Neuromol Med* 10: 59–66.
4. Kraft E. 2012 Cognitive function, physical activity, and aging: possible biological links, implications for multimodal interventions. *Neuropsychol Dev Cogn B Aging Neuropsychol Cogn.* 19(1-2):248–263.
5. Lista I, Sorrentino G. 2010 Biological mechanisms of physical activity in preventing cognitive decline. *Cell Mol Neurobiol* 30:493–503.
6. Angevaren M et al 2008 Physical activity and enhanced fitness to improve cognitive function in older people without known cognitive impairment. *Cochrane Database Syst Rev* 16: CD005381.
7. Voss MW et al 2012 The influence of aerobic fitness on cerebral white matter integrity and cognitive function in older adults: Results of a one-year exercise intervention. *Hum Brain Mapp.* 34:2972–2985.
8. Rhyu IJ et al 2010 Effects of aerobic exercise training on cognitive function and cortical vascularity in monkeys. *Neurosci* 167:1239–1248.
9. Secher NH et al 2008. Cerebral blood flow and metabolism during exercise: implications for fatigue. *J Appl Physiol.* 104:306–314.
10. Oudegeest-Sander MH et al 2013 Impact of physical fitness and daily energy expenditure on sleep efficiency in young and older humans. *Gerontology.* 59:8–16.
11. Fotuhi M et al 2012. Modifiable factors that alter the size of the hippocampus with ageing. *Nat Rev Neurol.* 8:189–202.
12. Woollett K, Maguire EA. 2011 Acquiring "the knowledge" of London's layout drives structural brain changes. *Curr. Biol.* 21: 2109–2114.
13. Mander BA et al 2013 Prefrontal atrophy, disrupted NREM slow waves and impaired hippocampal-dependent memory in aging. *Nat Neurosci.* 16:357–364.
14. Landsness EC et al 2009 Sleep-dependent improvement in visuomotor learning: a causal role for slow waves. Sleep; 32:1273–1284.

15. Naylor E et al 2000 Daily social and physical activity increases slow-wave sleep and daytime neuropsychological performance in the elderly. *Sleep*. 23:87–95.
16. Anderson C & Horne JA 2003 Pre-frontal cortex: links between low frequency delta EEG in sleep and neuro-psychological performance in healthy, older people. Psychophysiology, 40: 349–357.
17. Liao WC. 2002 Effects of passive body heating on body temperature and sleep regulation in the elderly: a systematic review. *Int J Nursing Studies*. 32: 803–810.
18. Mander BA et al 2015. ß-amyloid disrupts human NREM slow waves and related hippocampus-dependent memory consolidation. *Nat Neurosci*. Online advance publication.

13

REM Sleep: Food for Thought?

13.1 Phenomena

During our lifespan, REM sleep (REM) is most prolific 1–2 months before birth, occupying about half of the roughly 18 hours of the baby's daily sleep *in utero,* where REM probably provides essential, artificial stimulation for the developing brain in the absence of stimulation from the outside world. Soon after birth, with the baby being bombarded with real sensory stimulation, much of REM disappears, much more than non-REM, to be replaced by wakefulness. However, we adults retain a higher proportion of REM within sleep than do most other mammals; this is about 20 % of sleep compared with around 5–15 % for other mammals. One reason is that we adults resemble our infants more than any other ape. The retention of marked infant characteristics into adulthood, known as 'neoteny', is seen not only in our overall body shape and general anatomy, but in our remarkable ability to maintain a high degree of learning, even into old age, and for our cortex to continue adapting to new experiences and 'rewire' itself accordingly. This may help explain our relatively high amounts of REM in adulthood, to the extent that some of this REM still falls into the category of 'dispensability', like that

© The Editor(s) (if applicable) and The Author(s) 2016
J. Horne, *Sleeplessness,* DOI 10.1007/978-3-319-30572-1_13

of infants. Our adult REM predominates towards the end of a night's sleep, particularly as the usually last REM period (REMP, see hypnogram in Sect. 6.1) when sleep is less essential, and it is this last REMP which seems to be most dispensable.

REM is a complex and intriguing aspect of our sleep, and is not simply a platform for dreaming, especially as different parts of the brain are involved in REM and dreaming, and thus the two phenomena are not really synonymous. REM can appear in the absence of dreaming, or at least dreaming as we know it, especially when one considers the predominance of REM *in utero*.

The eponymous bursts of rapid eye movements (rems), characterising REM, which are absent from non-REM, typically appear every minute or so, lasting for about 15 seconds at a time, followed by a period of inactivity. Although rems are mostly 'saccadic', that is with the eyes moving together, darting from side to side as in wakefulness, these bursts are largely random, seeming to have little or nothing to do with the dream imagery. The rems per minute, known as 'REM density', are greatest during this last REMP, when dreams are also at their most vivid and intense. In fact, almost half of a whole night's worth of rems are found here, and it seems that this overall increased intensity in rems and dreaming may be a means for maintaining sleep as an alternative to wakefulness when there is little real need to wake up.

Interestingly, something similar to bursts of rems occurs concurrently within the ears during rems, called 'middle ear muscle activity' (MIMA), and is also found frequently during wakefulness to 'tone up hearing', and is comparable with 'pricking up one's ears'. Bursts of rems and MIMAs reflect the phasic component of REM, largely emanating from more 'basic' brain structures well below the cortex, where this is seen in the 'sub-cortical' EEG as bursts of pontine-geniculate-occipital (PGO) waves. These, together with rems and MIMAs seem to resemble an alerting response, in redirecting attention to a new stimulus.

I liken dreaming to the 'cinema of the mind', with what seems to be increasingly appealing dreams in successive REMPs, when dreams jump from one intriguing scene to another, maybe distracting us from waking. Dreams comprise a jumble of waking encounters, thoughts and emotions and, as Freud noted, 'we dream as we think', although I doubt whether attempts at dream interpretation are the 'royal road to unconsciousness' as he believed. As dreams are largely a mixture of personal experiences and thoughts, one must be sceptical about attempts by others to 'interpret' them, without knowledge of these experiences. Nevertheless, dreams are quite emotive, and may somehow help consolidate waking memories having particular emotional significance [1]. However, as we typically dream for about 90 minutes in total during the course of a night's sleep, and as much of dreaming seems to be nonsense, there is little opportunity to remember a dream unless we immediately wake up out of one, when little more than the previous few minutes can usually be recalled, even then, and is soon forgotten.

Recently, there has been much interest in what is known as the 'default mode network' of linked areas within the waking brain, largely identified by fMRI findings, with this network becoming most active during daydreaming [2] as well as during REM, but being less active during non-REM.

As noted earlier (Sect. 6.3), by extending sleep, as with a lie-in, and when not making up for previously lost sleep, the next, hitherto usually absent REMP (at around 7 hours' sleep), is even longer albeit not so intense in terms of REM density, suggesting that sleep has probably reached saturation. Nevertheless, if after waking up in the morning at the normal time, feeling refreshed and sleep satiated, we then decide to return to sleep, it is likely that another REM will reappear within 10 minutes of any sleep onset. This is known as a 'SOREMP'—sleep onset REM period. These otherwise absent examples of 'extra REM' seem to help sleep 'coast along', especially as this extra REM does not subtract from the ensuing night's amount of REM, nor change rem density. Thus, this particular REM seems quite surplus to requirements.

Another notable characteristic of REM is its associated atonia, a temporary paralysis of limb, trunk and facial muscles, preventing us from moving and thus physically enacting a dream. Sometimes, when woken up suddenly from a frightening nightmare, this atonia remains for a short while, often causing further alarm, especially as this also prevents speech. Known as 'isolated sleep paralysis', it is unlikely to be symptomatic of narcolepsy (see Sect. 9.5). This atonia may well have roles other than just safeguard the dreamer, as there may be a need for the brain to generate this physical movement during REM, to be blocked by the paralysis. Interestingly, if healthy sleepers are woken as soon as they enter REM, then get up and quietly walk around for about 15 minutes to return to sleep, and if this process is repeated whenever REM reappears that night, then there is little recovery of this lost REM ('REM rebound') the following night and, perhaps surprisingly, there is little by way of increased daytime sleepiness, cf. [3]. However, it is not known to what extent all this could be replicated into a second night and beyond. Nevertheless, substitution of REM by waking movement, with no subsequent REM rebound, has also been reported by several animal studies, cf. [3].

13.2 REM Wakefulness

REM is both a light and deep form of sleep, inasmuch that during REM we can hear what is going on around and unconsciously determine whether to wake up and respond to a noise or ignore it. This mechanism centres on the limbic system of the brain, most notably the amygdala, which in wakefulness is largely concerned with assessing the emotional significance of whatever is sensed. Throughout REM the amygdala remains active and can 'decide' whether a sound warrants a rapid awakening with full alertness or being blocked out. In this latter respect, REM seems to be a 'deep' form of sleep, allowing sleep to continue, and this is why a familiar train thundering by on a nearby railway is unlikely to cause an awakening during REM, whereas whispering a familiar name or the whimper of a child will cause an immediate awakening and rapid alertness. On the other hand, during SWS such arousals are largely a matter of the loudness of the sound rather than its meaning, requiring much more stimulation for an awakening, followed by grogginess and 'sleep inertia' lasting for several minutes (see Sect. 11.5). 'Light sleepers' are more reactive to sounds, especially during REM, and as they are more liable to wake up, so are they more likely to know they have been dreaming, unlike the 'sounder sleeper' who slumbers on, unable to remember their dreams.

Brain imaging using fMRI during REM also shows the activities of several other major brain areas to be similar to those of wakefulness, apart from the default mode network and the amygdala, which are in contrast with non-REM and quite different from SWS [4]. This similarity is also apparent in the EEGs of REM and relaxed wakefulness, where for many mammals REM is also known as 'paradoxical sleep' as the EEG appears to be like that of wakefulness, while the animal is clearly asleep.

With dreams often being emotional, and as REM can be a light sleep, it is surprising that we do not wake up more frequently from them. Despite such dream content, the actual emotional response is blocked, as there is no physiological arousal such as rapid rises in heart rate and blood pressure, as would happen in wakefulness. Although, if the dream develops into a nightmare and an awakening, these responses are triggered immediately. This blocking of responses is, again, largely under the control of the amygdala which, during wakefulness, also helps us to deal with threats and fears [5], as do the activities of other parts of the limbic system, notably the orbitofrontal region (see Fig. 10.1) of the frontal cortex which tones down more basic emotions into more acceptable ways [6]. The Appendix also gives examples of the effects on behaviour when this region is destroyed as a result of trauma, often leading to uninhibited and impaired social responses. The orbitofrontal region also happens to be active in REM, but not in non-REM.

Other key brain regions similarly active during both REM and wakefulness are the anterior cingulate cortex (ACC) and the hippocampus [4, 7]. In wakefulness the ACC helps resolve indecisions or conflicts between competing behavioural responses and in working out the payoffs, especially in terms of curiosity versus risk [8]. Inasmuch as curiosity can bring us into threatening situations, the amygdala and orbitofrontal cortex seem to contribute to the final decision on what to do. The hippocampus, mentioned earlier (Sect. 10.7), within the context of memory, not only is critical to the formation of long-term ('episodic') memories associated with personal events, experiences and related emotions, but also enables the navigating around our environment, with the creation of 'mental maps' (largely utilising hippocampal 'place neurones'), as well as with helping to integrate these memories.

In conjunction with other brain regions also active in REM, these mental maps might be created for the location of places having strong positive or negative emotional associations. Which brings me back to that atonia of REM, and the suppression of intended movements, as these might be integral to the creation of mental maps during REM. In wakefulness, locomotion is indeed integral to brain plasticity (see Sect. 12.1), including this mental mapping [9]. One might even speculate that the atonia of REM is somehow 'rehearsing' the physical movements between these more emotionally driven mapping points.

Whilst the role of REM in the more 'standard' forms of memory, outlined in Sect. 10.7, remains debatable [7], impressive evidence is accumulating that REM helps us cope with and stabilise the emotional memories of wakefulness [7, 10–13], not only in terms of what has happened recently, but also in preparation for the future. The term used is 'fear extinction', that is, the lessening of more fearful or apprehensive events, and maybe their locations, thus enabling one better able to deal with similar encounters in the future. However, in these respects there remains the puzzle of explaining the value of what must be the 'surplus' REM, seen in extended sleep and those SOREMPs.

Most antidepressant medicines reduce REM by at least 30 % (about 30 minute per night) [14, 15], with more extreme cases [16] of at least 50 % REM reductions for over 6 months. This absent REM seems largely replaced by interim wakefulness throughout the night, which may well be compensatory. It should be noted that this form of REM suppression is diffuse throughout the night, and not just a termination of the last REMP. Although there is some increase in REM ('REM rebound') when medication ceases, this only lasts a few days and, clearly, only represents a small fraction of the REM that has been lost. Interestingly, these long-term partial losses of REM do not seem to cause memory impairments.

As REM suppression is immediate when these medications are given, their beneficial effects on depression tend to take 2–4 weeks before becoming evident. So, the extent to which REM and dream loss are therapeutic remains a matter for conjecture, and it should be noted that most antidepressants are associated with changes to non-REM as well as with REM [15]. On the other hand, when severely depressed patients have their night sleep reduced to about 4 hours, thus losing the last one or two REMPs, there is often an immediate but temporary mood-improving effect the next day, which relapses on the return to normal sleep. But we cannot be certain that it is the loss of REM itself which is the key to this temporary mood improvement.

Certain dolphins and porpoises seem to have no REM whatsoever [17], and the sea lion has no REM for many weeks at a time when sleeping at sea [18], until the animal returns to land, when REM reappears, but even then there is no REM rebound. In both these cases, sleeping at sea necessitates frequent movement, with dolphins having to surface and breathe every few minutes, and sea lions needing to maintain stability with their flippers when sleeping on their backs, afloat. Possibly, these movements somehow substitute for REM and its atonia.

13.3 Appetite for REM

Many of the brain mechanisms underlying REM (unlike non-REM) are also in common with those controlling feeding behaviours [19]. This perhaps is not surprising due to the similarities between REM and wakefulness and that, until comparatively recent times, much of our wakefulness was spent seeking food. However, in doing this, there was also the risk of dangerous encounters needing to be avoided, but balanced against the attractiveness of the food source. Hence, there was also an element of fear, especially if this involved hunting and foraging in unfamiliar environments. I believe that REM still has a role to play in these respects, even today, with our safe and easy access to attractive foods.

Prominent amongst these common mechanisms is a group of the brain's 'neuropeptides' known as orexins [20], otherwise known as hypocretins, which not only affect REM but also influence emotional behaviour, appetite, and the assimilation of rewards. REM also seems able to suppress appetite, which might be particularly relevant to us, as our nocturnal sleep is quite long, usually following some hours after the last meal of the previous day, to the extent that the last part of our nocturnal sleep typically develops into a fasting state, when we would otherwise be hungry [21, 22], particularly during the usually final REMP of the night.

Thus, one might speculate that those habitual short sleepers (see Sect. 4.3), sleeping fewer than 5 hours a night, having lost this final REM, might have a heightened morning appetite, and the potential for a greater food consumption (if they chose to eat more), hence eventual obesity. However, I must be cautious here, as it will be remembered (Sect. 4.3) that their overall weight gain is both slow and small compared with the extent of what might be seen as the 'missing' REM. On the other hand, short-term studies of normally sleeping, non-obese volunteers report that acute reductions in REM lead to increases in hunger and greater subsequent carbohydrate consumption [23]. Interestingly, though, continuous intravenous infusion of glucose during a night's sleep, able to eliminate the early morning fast, prolongs REM rather than non-REM in the second half of sleep [24], and a high-carbohydrate meal eaten just before sleep, leading to higher blood glucose levels towards the end of sleep, also has the same effect [25]. Of course, these short-term experimental studies may well not be so relevant to the habitual very short sleeper; in addition, there is the issue of why some short sleepers are more liable to become obese, and others remain lean. Exactly how REM might interact with our feeding behaviour remains to be explored.

Although many REM-suppressing antidepressants (see Sect. 13.2) also lead to weight gain, this cannot solely be attributed to the lost REM, as other REM-suppressant medications do not affect body weight. However, as I mentioned, these medications do not simply remove this last REM, but have a more diffuse effect on REM throughout sleep.

Whether or not REM has 'anti-obesity' properties also remains an open matter, although there might well be subtle links with its influence on emotions. For example, our food preferences often have emotional associations in terms of like and dislike, even desire, as we eat palatable foods for their hedonic (gourmet) properties, independent of their nutritional status. The term 'forbidden fruit' comes to mind here. Interestingly, research outside the area of sleep [26] shows how excessive consumption of palatable food can affect the brain's reward mechanisms within the orbitofrontal cortex, amygdala and ACC. All of which also happen to be active in REM, as are the orexins. Moreover, as orexins have a role in converting sensory cues into reward-seeking behaviours, then so might REM [26].

Another perspective concerns those seasonal changes in daylight and darkness mentioned previously (Sects. 2.3 and 7.1) when, before the advent of artificial lighting, people would have been likely to have adjusted their sleep duration according to the seasonal changes in daylight and its implications in terms of food availability, and with the different demands on wakefulness in foraging for food. By affecting sleep duration this would have a particular impact on the preponderance of REM at the end of sleep. That is, one might speculate that with increasing summer daylight, to facilitate more productive foraging, the final REMP might disappear in order to allow for more food collection in preparation for food shortages during the winter, when sleep would be longer. Moreover, the temporary summer loss of this REMP, resulting in a potentially enhanced appetite coupled with a greater abundance of food, might well encourage overeating, and lead to 'protective obesity' in preparation for the leaner times of the winter when these fat reserves would be utilised.

Furthermore, as we are so dependent on our eyes and poor at seeing in the dark, there was little point, then, in waking up before dawn during the long winter nights. Thus to prevent the overnight fast from causing premature awakening during the winter, any role REM has in suppressing appetite and feeding behaviour, by prolonging sleep until dawn, would be advantageous.

13.4 Summary

The case is made that our final REM period retains a 'dispensability' (as in infancy), able to be substituted by wakefulness (without a REM rebound) when pressures of wakefulness increase. Alternatively, when sleeping in a safe environment with, for example, food being plentiful and we have 'time to spare', sleep can be extended further, with extra REM.

REM is similar to wakefulness in a variety of ways, and resembles exploratory behaviours involving stimulation, curiosity and aspects of emotions, quite possibly including mental mapping of places having 'emotional connotations'. These are characteristics quite different to those of non-REM. REM particularly seems to regulate waking emotional tone, especially by dampening fear responses. In effect, REM appears to be preparing us for forthcoming wakefulness, rather than acting as a recovery process from prior wakefulness, as seems to be the case with SWS. REM may well be linked to feeding behaviours, given their common brain mechanisms, with REM seeming to act as an appetite suppressant, especially during the latter part of our nocturnal sleep, which typically develops into a fast. One explanation integrating all these findings and for REM being 'wake-like', is that in older times our wakefulness was preoccupied in searching for food, which necessitated balancing curiosity against the potential for encountering danger with its implicit fear. As we also select foods for their hedonic (emotional) values, REM may even be integral to developing food preferences and avoidances (dislikes).

For most of us today life is fairly safe. This, together with the abundance of risk-free food, can lead to a relatively rapid feeling of satiation, which could be 'confusing' for these underlying brain mechanisms affecting appetite and the need to forage for food. That REM might be involved in regulating food intake this may even promote obesity in some (but not all) short sleepers who may have 'lost' their last REMP and even seek needless food for 'emotional' reasons. On the other hand, as relatively little of our wakefulness is required for finding food then, today, these exploratory attributes of REM can be directed to other aspects of waking life.

In effect, there is much about REM which is intriguing, is largely overlooked and remains little explored, unlike dreaming, which may well be just the 'icing on this REM cake'. That is, dreaming helps entertain the sleeping brain and maybe distract it from waking up when wakefulness is unproductive, by providing even more novel and engrossing stimulation towards the end of sleep, as reflected by a greater intensity of rems and dreaming, to further feed our curiosity. Thus, REM helps to keep the sleeping brain in 'quiet readiness' for wakefulness. Apart from protecting the dreamer, the accompanying paralysis (atonia) may also be a 'substitute for locomotion', and to these ends REM might well help create those 'mental maps' of the location of waking 'emotional' encounters, perhaps originally more oriented towards food sources, and thus helping us to anticipate what to avoid or be attracted to.

Thus, the 'ideal amount of sleep' will depend on these various waking pressures underlying the propensity for REM, which is able to adapt, without necessarily incurring sleep debt if REM is forfeited, and without REM rebounds. Nevertheless, the likely interactions between daylight, artificial light and the accompanying circadian influences on sleep (especially REM) add to this intrigue behind feeding and other exploratory behaviours potentially linked to REM.

Much needs to be understood about this still enigmatic form of sleep, which has to be studied beyond the laboratory, in real-world 'ecological' settings that incorporate a broader repertoire of human behaviour outside the usual remit of sleep research. Indeed, maybe it is REM rather than sleep itself, which Shakespeare referred to as the *"chief nourisher in life's feast"*. Macbeth (2.2.46-51).

References

1. Blagrove M et al 2011, Assessing the dream-lag effect for REM and NREM stage 2 dreams. *PLoS ONE* 6, e26708.
2. Mason MF et al, 2007, Wandering minds, the default network and stimulus-independent thought. *Science* 315: 393–395.
3. Horne J. 2013 Why REM sleep? Clues beyond the laboratory in a more challenging world. *Biol Psychol*. 92:152–168.
4. Dang-Vu TT et al 2010, Functional neuroimaging insights into the physiology of human sleep. *Sleep* 33:1589–1603.
5. Bickart KC et al 2011 Amygdala volume and social network size in humans. *Nature Neurosci* 14:163–164.
6. Jacobs RAH 2012 The amygdala, top-down effects, and selective attention to features. *Neurosci Biobehav Rev* 36:2069–2084.
7. Rasch B, Born J 2013 About sleep's role in memory *Physiol Rev*. 93:681–766.
8. Jepma M et al 2012 Neural mechanisms underlying the induction and relief of perceptual curiosity. *Front Behav Neurosci* 6, 5 Epub.
9. Kempermann G et al 2010 Why and how physical activity promotes experience-induced brain plasticity. *Frontiers Neurosci*. 4, Article 189, 1–9.
10. Vandekerckhove M, Cluydts R., 2010, The emotional brain and sleep, an intimate relationship. *Sleep Med Rev* 14, 219–226.
11. Van der Helm E et al 2011. REM sleep depotentiates amygdala activity to previous emotional experiences. *Curr Biol* 21: 2029–2032.
12. Gujar N et al 2011, A role for rem sleep in recalibrating the sensitivity of the human brain to specific emotions. *Cerebral Cortex* 21:115–123.
13. Baran B et al 2012 Processing of emotional memory over sleep. *J Neurosci*. 32:1035–1042.

14. Göder R et al 2011, Sleep and cognition at baseline and the effects of REM sleep diminution after 1 week of antidepressive treatment in patients with depression. *J Sleep Res* 20: 544–551.

15. Steiger A, Kimura M, 2010, Wake and sleep EEG provide biomarkers in depression. *J Psychiat Res.* 44:42–52.

16. Landolt HP, de Boer LP 2001, Effect of chronic phenelzine treatment on REM sleep, report of three patients. *Neuropsychopharm* 25: S63–S67.

17. Siegel JM 2009, Sleep viewed as a state of adaptive inactivity. *Nature Rev Neurosci* 10:747–753.

18. Lyamin OI., 2002, Sleep and wakefulness in the southern sea lion. *Behav Brain Res* 128: 29–38.

19. Kolling N et al 2012 Neural mechanisms of foraging. *Science.*; 336: 95–98.

20. Sakurai T 2014 The role of orexin in motivated behaviours *Nat Rev Neurosci.* 15:719–31.

21. Horne JA. 2009 REM sleep, energy balance and optimal foraging. Neurosci Biobehav Rev 33: 466–474.

22. Hayes AL, Xu F, Babineau D, Patel SR. 2011 Sleep duration and circulating adipokine levels. Sleep; 34:147–152.

23. Shechter A et al 2012 Alterations in sleep architecture in response to experimental sleep curtailment are associated with signs of positive energy balance. *Am J Physiol - Reg Integ Comp Physiol.* 303:R883–R889.

24. Benedict C et al 2009 Early morning rise in hypothalamic-pituitary-adrenal activity: a role for maintaining the brain's energy balance. *Psychoneuroendocrinol*; 34:55–62.

25. Porter JM, Horne JA. 1981 Bed-time food supplements and sleep: effects of different carbohydrate levels. *Electroenceph Clin Neurophysiol.*51: 26–33.

26. Kenny PJ. 2011 Reward mechanisms in obesity: new insights and future directions. Neuron 69:664–679.

14

Overview

Despite beliefs about 'societal insomnia', of a widespread sleep debt and its being linked to obesity, cardiovascular disease and other disorders, *Sleeplessness* has maintained that our sleep duration has changed little over the last hundred or so years and that these apparent adverse health effects are often overstated. If for argument's sake we slept for longer, then why might this be considered as 'better' sleep, and presumably 'good' for our health, given those poorer living conditions, greater social deprivation, more illness and a shorter life expectancy? Sleepwise, were those really the 'good old days'. Why not argue that this apparent longer sleep merely compensated for the austerity?

Sleep is more adaptable than is generally thought, more so perhaps before the advent of the electric light and the industrial age, when seasonal changes in daylight and the accompanying changes to the availability of different foods and other waking pressures would have impacted on the time for daily sleep.

By asking people, today, 'would you like more sleep?' encourages positive answers, maybe indicative of sleep debt, but fails to discriminate between actual sleep need versus a desire for just sleeping for pleasure. We can eat to excess without hunger, merely from a 'hearty appetite',

© The Editor(s) (if applicable) and The Author(s) 2016
J. Horne, *Sleeplessness*, DOI 10.1007/978-3-319-30572-1_14

and drink socially for enjoyment, without thirst. Similarly, we can sleep in excess of its need, just for gratification or out of boredom, reflecting an 'appetite for sleep' rather than a 'sleep hunger', an actual sleep need.

Definitions of 'habitually short sleep' are often vague and confused by 'time in bed'. Besides, judging sleep merely by its length ignores the importance of its quality, as hour by hour a night's sleep is not equivalent in terms of recuperation, which declines as sleep progresses. All too easily overlooked are the benefits of the daytime nap, most efficient sleepwise.

Human behaviour being what it is, the various paradoxes and misperceptions accompanying actual ('primary' or 'psychophysiological') insomnia have never really changed historically, with it also often a form of 'overwakefulness' rather than a lack of sleep. Moreover, our striving for an unbroken night's sleep, as is the custom nowadays, might even be somewhat 'unnatural' in being a relatively recent habit.

Interactions between the circadian clock and sleep provided further insights into sleep duration, further pointing to the adaptability of sleep according to these external circumstances and pressures, not forgetting individual differences between larks and owls. All of which suggested that the intriguing, recent concept of 'social jet lag', rather similar to sleep debt, may not be so problematic as is claimed, unlike the other issues associated with shift work and actual jet lag where some practical advice is given.

Many 'statistically significant findings' relating to the adverse effects on health of sleep debt are of questionable real clinical importance, as are claims of 'short sleep' being a cause of obesity, type 2 diabetes, hypertension and depression. Neither by extending sleep, even by using sleeping tablets to counteract these presumed effects, are there likely to be improvements when compared with a better diet, more exercise and a less stressful lifestyle. Laboratory studies of acute sleep restriction, causing 'pre-diabetic-like' symptoms in healthy adults, apparently endorsing the adverse effects of short sleep, seem to be too extreme and intolerable in terms of heightened sleepiness and risk of serious accidents.

Despite claims to the contrary, sleep duration in children has also changed little over the last century, even improved in some countries. Similar conclusions on the extent to which sleep debt relates to obesity apply to both adult and children. Adolescence brings its own essential changes to sleep, of course, accompanied by the debatable 'need versus desire' for lie-ins and whether school start times should be delayed.

Sleepiness was viewed from various perspectives. Firstly, it was distinguished from 'tiredness', often seen with insomnia as a weariness not necessarily caused by insomnia, and not easily treated by sleeping tablets, but more effectively by psychological therapies. Secondly, inasmuch as sleepiness feeds on monotony and boredom, readily appearing under these circumstances in its mild form, it is most detectable by sensitive albeit tedious tests and might be seen as a further sign of sleep debt. But these otherwise excellent tests can be oversensitive in uncovering a level of sleepiness that would not exist under usual living conditions and is seen as situational or 'appetitive sleepiness'. Thirdly, a topic with many ramifications is our ability to be aware of our own sleepiness which might be seen to be poor, thus necessitating these tests for its detection. However, given a few minutes to relax, in a manner comparable with these measures, then we can more easily notice it in ourselves but then fail to recognise the risks, particularly in continuing to drive in this state. Finally, and in contrast was the persistent and severe sleepiness seemingly 'noticed but unrealised' by sufferers from major sleep disorders, such as chronic obstructive sleep apnoea syndrome.

Sleep not only relieves sleepiness but has other less obvious, vital benefits for the hard-working, waking cerebral cortex, especially the frontal region, largely responsible for more subtle behaviours, collectively called 'executive function'. However, not all of sleep is equivalent in terms of this cortical recovery, as slow wave sleep (SWS), especially its low frequency EEG component, particularly reflects this recovery, predominant in early sleep, more so in the frontal area.

Impairments to executive behaviours caused by little or no sleep are not so apparent within a laboratory setting, and were overlooked until recently; they are more readily evident outside the laboratory under real-life, more demanding conditions, especially when we are confronted by unexpected events, and having to 'think out of the box' with risky decision-making, as can occur with extended wakefulness during an initial night shift. Such effects are also to be seen if we are suddenly awoken from SWS, as the frontal area requires some minutes to become fully engaged with reality. A historical account of the evolution the wider understanding of this crucial brain region, outside the topic of sleep, is given in the Appendix.

Cognition is inseparable from physical activity, and together the two help offset cortical ageing, by stimulating cortical plasticity, seemingly mostly facilitated by SWS. All one may well need for enhancing this brainwork and thus more SWS, is a comfortable pair of shoes, a sense of exploration fired by curiosity and the habit to get out and about somewhere new, to meet, greet, engage and interact with others and one's surroundings. Routine, monotonous exercise alone is probably not sufficient.

Whereas SWS largely consolidates the previous day's events, REM seems more oriented towards preparing us for wakefulness, especially with its abundance towards the end of sleep, and its similarities with wakefulness. REM's accompanying dreaming probably acts more as a time-filler, occupying the sleeping brain, able to further extend sleep when pressures for wakefulness are low. REM and wakefulness can switch with each other, at least towards the end of sleep. Inasmuch as REM also has brain mechanisms in common with feeding behaviour and appetite control, together with its role in modifying emotions, it may even help with the balancing of 'fear against curiosity' in anticipated future waking encounters, and even affect our desirability of certain foods.

Sleeplessness began by trying to allay various concerns of those with insomnia, notably, about how much sleep is really needed, and that what is seen as 'missing' sleep might even be an opportunity for a more enjoyable wakefulness. This is not to deny that insomnia is distressing, but with these further insights I hope *Sleeplessness* might provide for a greater peace of mind about sleep, even lead to better sleep.

Appendix: Frontal Assault

Early Traumas

We owe much to our understanding of the functions of the frontal cortex to a memorable event involving Phineas Gage, who in September 1848 was working on a Vermont railroad when a 43 inch, 13 lb tamping rod accidentally shot out of a blast hole, hit him in the face and destroyed part of his frontal cortex. He survived to live a somewhat different but reasonable life, ending up as a long-distance stagecoach driver in Chile. However, his behaviour became more bizarre and his personality changed towards what his physician, Dr John Martyn Harlow, referred to as his becoming a "ne'er-do-well braggadocio". Dr Harlow himself enjoyed considerable fame and fortune as a result of Gage's calamity, and wrote much about his patient, including a 20-page article, eight years after Gage's death [1]. The salient point, here, is that despite his losing a substantive part of his frontal cortex, which apparently had little by way of major effect on his subsequent behaviour, for the next hundred years it gave the scientific world the impression that this brain region was rather redundant.

In fact, there are many overlooked, rather similar accounts predating this event, of people losing significant portions of this same brain region, and surviving with little apparent ill effect. Many of these traumas were

© The Editor(s) (if applicable) and The Author(s) 2016
J. Horne, *Sleeplessness*, DOI 10.1007/978-3-319-30572-1

from exploding muskets, caused by the gun's breech being overloaded with gunpowder, then backfiring into the owner's forehead positioned just behind the breech during aiming and firing. Summaries of these and several remarkable other cases can be found in the British Medical Journal of 1853, in an editorial entitled, *"Cases of recovery after loss of portions of the brain"* (29 April, pp. 375–376), with the earliest account coming from the Battle of Waterloo (1815) of a case of a musket ball entering a soldier's forehead and lodging within his brain. Seemingly, he fully recovered from these symptoms, obeyed orders to the letter (note this), rejoined the army and lived for another twelve years, eventually dying of TB.

A few years later, a letter by Dr John Edmonson, in the *Edinburgh Medical and Surgical Journal* of April 1822 (p. 199), told of a 15-year-old soldier who was wounded by the bursting breech of a small cannon. Shrapnel blew through his forehead, leaving thirty-two pieces of bone and metal that were removed from the frontal part of his brain, together with *"a tablespoon of cerebral substance ... portions of brain were also discharged at three dressings"*. The account went on to say *"at no period were there any symptoms referable to this injury ... during the time that the brain was discharged he is reported as giving correct answers to questions put to him, and as being perfectly rational."* After three months he was reported to be in perfect health, "having suffered no derangement of his mental capacities".

The year 1827 saw a report by a Dr Rogers in the *Medico-Chirurgical Transactions*, where a young man received what eventually turned out to be severe frontal brain injuries from a musket breech explosion, initially thought not be serious, as he rapidly recovered, although three weeks later a 3 inch, 3 ounce breech pin was removed from within his cranial cavity, and four months later he was reported to be *"perfectly cured"*. Case number 14 described in this BMJ editorial, was of an exploding breech pin penetrating 1½ inches into the forehead, making a hole ¾ inch in diameter, resulting in an *"escape of cerebral substance"*. But *"no severe symptoms occurred, and recovery took place in less than 24 days"*.

In 1853, a Dr De Barbe reported in the *Gazette des Hôpitaux Chaumes*, that a soldier hit by pieces of the breech that penetrated the forehead, was still able to search for other fragments of his gun (as to why he did this we don't know) and then walk some distance to the hospital, where, *"a piece of the gun was removed, a spoonful of cerebral matter escaped".* Moreover, and note, *"there was no disturbance of intellect, nor of the senses, nor speech throughout the progress of the case. On the twelfth day the patient was discharged."*

Given these deep penetrating injuries, it is surprising that the casualties did not die of wound infection. But one advantage of gunpowder is that it is also a strong antiseptic, which soldiers would sprinkle on battle wounds. As the foreheads of these victims were probably fortuitously coated with gunpowder dust, before penetration by what would have been a sterile piece of breech, the risk of infection was reduced. Thankfully, though, by around 1860 most of these injuries disappeared as did the musket, having been replaced by the rifle and all-metal cartridges.

A more detailed account of a civilian injury can be seen in another issue of the BMJ, in an article entitled, *"Case of recovery after compound fracture of the frontal bone and loss of cerebral substance",* by George Mallet (15 July 1853, p. 610). Mr R Booth, a 60-year-old stone mason, was struck on the head by the handle of a rapidly rotating windlass. He was knocked out and then carried by his fellow labourers back to his house, where his situation was considered hopeless by a passing "medical gentleman". Nevertheless, the next day he was still alive, and his GP (Dr Mallet), was called, to find that Booth was still "insensible", having sustained a compound fracture of the entire breadth of frontal bone, with a large piece driven into the brain; *"a very considerable quantity of the cerebral matter was adherent to the adjoining parts … the quantity of the brain lost could not be accurately estimated, but it was not thought to be less than from one to two tablespoonfuls"* (p. 610).

With the assistance of a medical friend, Dr Mallet proceeded to remove pieces of the bone that were deeply embedded into the cortex. Twelve such bone fragments were removed, and *"still the man remained quite insensible to our operations; but on the extraction of the thirteenth, the last, which was a larger piece and more deeply imbedded than the others, he started up in bed and uttered—no doubt from his accustomed habit, and quite unconscious of what had been going on—an oath".* Dressings were applied and Booth was left until the next morning, when Dr Mallet found him *"quite sensible and exhibiting no unfavourable symptoms".* The only medication he then received was castor oil, for his bowels.

Three months later Dr Mallet reported that Booth had walked three miles to the surgery, and that *"pulsations of the brain were seen immediately under the newly formed skin ... his intellect, as far as I could judge, was unimpaired; and the muscular power not at all paralysed. I never saw him afterwards"*.

The Next 100 Years

Until well into the 1950s, it was still thought that this brain region was of little real use, with its loss merely causing a 'blunting of the emotions', to the extent that its surgical separation from the rest of the cortex might well be of benefit to those with various mental disorders, including depression. Amongst the first to see this potential was the Portuguese neurologist Dr Egas Moniz who, in 1935, demonstrated that surgery on the frontal lobes could easily be accomplished in sedated but non-anaesthetised psychiatric patients. Over the following ten years he refined his techniques for 'frontal lobectomy' and for this work he was awarded the Nobel Prize for Medicine and Physiology in 1949.

By 1937 the practice had spread rapidly, especially in the USA, regardless of there being no objective clinical evaluations akin to the 'randomised placebo controlled trials' of today. Despite mounting opposition from many psychiatrists, who viewed 'psychosurgery' as replacing psychiatric illness with brain damage, lobotomies became even more popular in the USA during the Second World War, largely to deal with a disquieting increase in psychiatric cases, as around half of the public hospital beds were occupied by the long-stay mentally ill. It set the scene for Dr Walter Freeman who, in 1946, invented the 'ice pick lobotomy' (sic); a procedure requiring only a kitchen 'ice pick' and a rubber mallet. Using only local anaesthesia, Freeman would deftly hammer the ice pick through the thin skull of his patients, just above the tear duct, and then sweep the pick back and forth to sever connections in his 'transorbital procedure'. Leaving no apparent scars, it was a far simpler technique than that of Moniz, involving having to drill untidy burr holes in the skull. Freeman would even line up patients for 'surgery' in his own office.

The crudeness of his method in violently projecting a piece of steel through the skull and mashing up the frontal cortex has to be likened to those earlier exploding musket breeches propelled through the forehead. Nevertheless, his technique was seen as a great advance in neurosurgery, able to be performed in mental hospitals lacking surgical facilities. Such was Freeman's enthusiasm that he eventually travelled around the USA in his own van, which he called his "lobotomobile", demonstrating the procedure in numerous medical centres, even in hotel rooms. Thankfully, he eventually lost his licence to practice when he killed a patient who was seeing him for her third such procedure.

Lost Souls

Despite reports, even from the late 1930s, of lifeless, unreactive individuals whose personalities were forever destroyed, such outcomes were largely ignored for many more years. Even in 1949 a notable paper [2] lamented *"these patients are not only no longer distressed by their mental conflicts but also seem to have little capacity for any emotional experiences—pleasurable or otherwise. They are described by the nurses and the doctors, over and over, as dull, apathetic, listless, without drive or initiative, flat, lethargic, placid and unconcerned, childlike, docile, needing pushing, passive, lacking in spontaneity, without aim or purpose, preoccupied and dependent."* Nevertheless, by the 1950s well over 50,000 Americans had undergone lobotomies of one sort or another, performed on patients with severe obsessive-compulsive and hypochondriac states, intractable back-pain and migraine, and on children as young as thirteen for 'delinquent behaviour'. There are even reports of it being used on depressed housewives who had 'lost their zeal for domestic work' and, in other countries, on political dissidents.

In the UK, the more tempered technique of 'prefrontal leucotomy' was adopted, again, mostly within psychiatric hospitals. After drilling a small burr hole above the eye orbit a pencil-sized 'leucotome' was inserted, with wire loops deployed to sever parts of the frontal lobe. And that was that—all over in about 10 minutes. In 1961, a follow-up [3] on 9,284 UK patients reported that 41 % had recovered or were greatly improved, 28 % were minimally improved, 25 % showed no change, 2 % had become worse and 4 % had died. Seemingly, patients with depression showed the best effect, with 63 % improving. But it was not until powerful neuroleptic medicines, such as chlorpromazine, appeared in the mid-1950s that lobotomies fell out of fashion.

We now know that people with frontal damage can usually undertake normal everyday routines, carry out orders, and appear 'normal'. However, they are more apathetic, inflexible to change, lose spontaneity, have poor short-term ('working') memory, less insight into their own performance, and are unlikely to engage in meaningful and interactive conversations, that is have a dialogue. Additional damage to the very front of the frontal cortex, the 'orbitofrontal cortex' above the eyes (see Fig. 10.1), due to those impacts to the forehead just described, would typically cause more risky, rude and bawdy behaviour, excessive swearing, rash decision-making, hypersexuality, childish humour, a disregard for normal social conventions, as well as a loss of empathy towards others, inappropriate interpersonal behaviours and even compulsive gambling. However, much has still yet to be understood about what other functions this complex brain area undertakes [4].

Imagine then, those brain injured nineteenth century musketeers who subsequently lived uneventful lives of routine who, in viewing their treating doctor with much deference and respect, would hardly engage in casual conversation or reveal these other behaviours. Neither would those early doctors be sufficiently familiar enough with their patients to spot these more subtle changes in behaviour. Thus, for all intents and purposes, these walking wounded could return to the ranks, where not only would their newfound bawdiness be admired by their mates, but they would be suitably dutiful to fight another day.

References

1. Harlow JM 1868. Recovery from the passage of an iron bar through the head. *Publications of the Massachusetts Medical Society*, 2: 327–347.
2. Hoffman JL 1949 Clinical observations concerning schizophrenic patients treated by prefrontal leucotomy *New Engl J Med.* 241:233–6.
3. Tooth GC, Newton, MP 1961 *Leucotomy in England and Wales, 1942–54.* London: HMSO.
4. Stalnaker TA et al. 2015 *What the orbitofrontal cortex does not do.* Nature Neurosci, 18: 620–627.

Index

© The Editor(s) (if applicable) and The Author(s) 2016
J. Horne, *Sleeplessness*, DOI 10.1007/978-3-319-30572-1

Printed by Printforce, the Netherlands